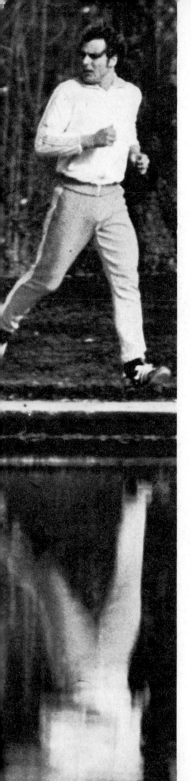

Charles B. Corbin
Kansas State University

Linus J. Dowell
Texas A & M University

Ruth Lindsey
California State University—Long Beach

Homer Tolson
Texas A & M University

Third Edition

Concepts in Physical Education

with Laboratories and Experiments

wcb

Wm. C. Brown Company Publishers
Dubuque, Iowa

Book Team

Ed Bowers, Jr., Publisher
Don Rivers, Editor
Marilyn Phelps, Designer
Patricia L. A. Hendricks, Production Editor

Wm. C. Brown Company Publishers

Wm. C. Brown, President
Larry W. Brown, Executive Vice-President
Lawrence E. Cremer, Vice-President, Director, College Division
Richard C. Crews, Publisher
Ray Deveaux, National Sales Manager
John Graham, National Marketing Manager
Roger Meyer, Director, Production/Manufacturing
John Carlisle, Assistant Vice-President, Production Division
Ruth Richard, Manager, Production-Editorial Department
David Corona, Design Director

PHYSICAL EDUCATION

Consulting Editor
Aileene Lockhart
Texas Woman's University

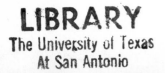

Contents

Preface

This text is designed primarily for an introductory course in physical education at the college level. New up-to-date material has been added to this third edition in an attempt to provide the reader with the best scientific evidence in the area of physical education. Though it covers many areas in the broad field of physical education, this book primarily deals with the specific areas of physical activity, exercise, health, physical fitness, skill learning, and body mechanics.

An outline format is used to give the reader a concise and factual presentation with regard to the HOW, WHAT, and WHY of physical activity and exercise. Discussion has been kept to a minimum; bibliographies, suggested readings, and extensive documentation are provided for the reader who wishes to further pursue a specific topic.

There are twenty concepts and forty accompanying laboratory exercises that are appropriate for both men and women. In an attempt to make the text materials as easy to use as possible, all self-evaluation materials, exercise programs, and laboratory information is incorporated into one lab section of the text. In the lab section, some material is meant to be torn out to be handed in as lab reports. However, where possible exercises, rating charts, and other similar information are provided on separate sheets from lab reports so that this information can be kept in the book for future reference. The reader is encouraged to keep the book for future use in selecting exercise programs and for doing self-evaluations. An understanding and appreciation of the information presented in these pages should provide the foundation for an intelligent selection of activities and health practices to aid the individual in leading a useful and productive life.

A comprehensive Instructor's Manual is available to teachers who use the text in their classes. It includes suggestions for organizing the classes, grading, lecture outlines, and laboratory instructions, as well as suggested supplementary activities. A master set of illustrations suitable for transparencies is available to accompany the lectures.

The authors wish to extend a special thanks to Robert Clayton, Colorado State University; Melvin Ezell, Jr., The Citadel; John Hayes, Northern Illinois University; R. G. Lawman, Miami Dade Junior College-South Campus; Alfred Leister, Mercer County Community College; Mary Rice, Glassboro State College; Roberta Stokes, Miami Dade Junior College-South campus; and Dennis Wilson, Auburn University, for their important advice and suggestions for improving this third edition of the book.

A Note to the Reader

This book is not exactly like other textbooks you may have used in the past. To make the book as easy to use as possible, we have organized the book in a unique way.

First, the book is written in a outline format. For this reason, the book does not read like most texts. However, the information will be useful and precise. Secondly, references are listed to support the facts presented in the text. While we do not expect you to look up each reference, we do want you to know where to look for more information about the facts that are presented if you want additional knowledge.

Another important feature of the book is the "tear out" lab sheets. These sheets have been perforated so that you can hand them in to your instructor, if requested. We have made sure that important testing or exercise information will not be torn out with these sheets, because we feel that you will want to keep this information for future use. Finally, special "program" appendixes are included at the end of the book. Many different exercise programs are presented in this section, and, in each case, the advantages and disadvantages of the various exercises are discussed.

This book is intended to help you make important decisions about your own personal exercise program and your personal physical fitness for now and for the rest of your life. We trust that you will find the book interesting and useful.

The Authors

Being physically educated is an important part of one's total education.

Introduction

Concept 1

Being physically educated is an important part of one's total education.

Introduction

Automation and technology have freed many people from the exhausting physical labor required of earlier generations. The fatiguing physical labor of the farmer and manual laborer is not part of the normal daily activity pattern for the majority of individuals. However, the need for sound physical and mental health and physical fitness, which result from regular exercise, is still quite necessary for every individual. In addition, the "free time" that has been made available to the average individual has created a need for the development of recreational skills that can be used for a lifetime. The physically educated man and woman must be able to make intelligent decisions concerning health, physical fitness, and recreational pursuits and to recognize the role of exercise and physical activity in daily life. Though the average man and woman in our society do not get adequate physical activity, a recent survey conducted by the President's Council on Physical Fitness and Sport indicated that more than 90 percent of American citizens felt that . . . "people should have physical education in school." (220)

The Facts

Too many Americans suffer from "hypokinetic diseases."

A "hypokinetic disease" is a disease that relates to or is caused by the lack of regular physical activity. (167) These diseases of sedentary man include coronary heart disease, high blood pressure, low back pain, and obesity, to name just a few. While recent advances in modern medicine have been quite effective in eliminating infectious diseases, the degenerative diseases, characterized by sedentary or "take-it-easy" living, have increased. Heart disease is the leading cause of death in the United States, with one man in five and slightly fewer women being stricken before the age of fifty. (90) As many as 45 percent of Americans are considered to be obese (133), and low back pain is a leading medical complaint. (165, 97) Apparently, the onset of these diseases can begin in youth. The fact that too many American children score poorly on tests of physical fitness (102) suggests that the future will not see a reduced rate of "hypokinetic disease" in our culture.

Regular physical activity and exercise can reduce the risk of "hypokinetic disease."

Scientific evidence, including a long-range study of an entire community, shows that people who exercise regularly are less likely to have degenerative diseases. (145) In fact, the death rate among active people is approximately one-half that of those who exhibit an inactive life-style. (102) At least one of every five adult Americans has been advised by a physician to get involved in regular exercise. (220)

Many people do not recognize the relationship between "hypokinetic disease" and physical inactivity.

A recent study shows that 45 percent of all adult Americans (about 49 million people) do not participate in physical activity for exercise. Those who *do not* exercise regularly believe they get enough exercise! Interestingly, those who report that they participate in regular exercise are more likely to feel that they do not get enough exercise for their own good health. (220)

Physical activity, including games and sports, is an enjoyable way to spend one's leisure hours.

Labor Department statistics indicate that in the past century the average workweek has been reduced by about thirteen hours, netting the average person 675 more hours of free time annually. With vacations and holidays added, the typical worker has 800 more free hours per year. (125) Increased sales of boats, campers, and other lifetime sports equipment indicate that many Americans are enjoying their leisure through participation in these activities.

Efficient movement is essential to effective living.

Although movement is unique to each individual, there are general guidelines for the efficient performance of movement skills used in the course of daily living. Whether it be walking, working on an assembly line, or performing household chores, learning to move efficiently is important to avoid strain and conserve energy.

The physical skills that an individual learns should be applicable for recreational use for a lifetime.

Most American adults who do exercise regularly indicate that they walk, ride a bike, jog, or swim. Among sports, bowling, golf, swimming, and tennis are the most popular. (220) Every individual should possess skills in "lifetime" sports and should have a knowledge of general exercises that could be used to promote health and physical fitness.

An individual should know WHY physical activity and exercise are important as well as HOW to perform various exercises and physical activities.

A study by Brunner (30) showed that 63 percent of the adults he interviewed felt the exercises and activities they learned as children and young adults were not applicable for use as adults. A more recent study indicates that very few people participate in competitive sports as adults. (71) Many of those interviewed in these studies have indicated that it would be desirable to learn WHY exercise is important to every adult so that the decision as to WHAT to do and HOW to do it would be more meaningful.

The choice of exercises and physical activities should be unique to each individual.

No two people are alike; therefore, physical activity patterns should be based on individual needs and interests. The decision concerning choice of exercise and physical activities should be made only after carrying out the following five steps:

1. Assess current health and physical fitness status to determine individual needs.
2. Examine current interests. (Physical activity should be enjoyable.)
3. Acquire a knowledge and understanding of the values of physical activity and exercise.
4. Determine which activities will best meet individual needs and interests.
5. Acquire skill and knowledge in the activities selected.

"Physical fitness is not only one of the most important keys to a healthy body; it is also the basis of dynamic and creative activity."

John F. Kennedy

Physical Fitness

Concept 2

"Physical fitness is not only one of the most important keys to a healthy body; it is also the basis of dynamic and creative activity." (155)

Introduction

Physical fitness has been defined by many people in several different ways. It is difficult to adequately define such a complex human characteristic. One point of consensus is that physical fitness is a desirable quality to possess. The following information is presented not only to aid the individual in developing a personal definition of physical fitness, but also to aid in developing a better understanding of the nature of physical fitness.

Health-Related Fitness Terms

Body Composition—The relative make-up of the body in muscle, fat, bone, and other vital parts.

Cardiovascular Fitness—The ability of the circulatory and respiratory systems to supply fuel (most importantly, oxygen) during sustained physical activity.

Flexibility—The range of motion available in a joint.

Muscular Endurance—The ability of muscle groups to exert external force for many repetitions or successive exertions.

Strength—The amount of external force that a muscle can exert.

Skill-Related Fitness Terms

Agility—The ability to rapidly change position of the entire body in space with speed and accuracy.

Balance—The maintenance of equilibrium while stationary or moving.

Coordination—The ability to use the senses, such as sight or hearing, together with the body parts in performing motor tasks smoothly and accurately.

Power—The ability to transfer energy into force at a fast rate of speed.

Reaction Time—The time elapsed between stimulation and the beginning of the reaction to it.

Speed—The ability to perform a movement in a short period of time.

The Facts

1. *Physical fitness is a part of total fitness.*

   Aspects of total fitness include emotional, social, spiritual, and mental as well as physical.

   Physical fitness consists of many components each of which is specific in nature. (142)

2. Physical fitness is a combination of several aspects rather than a single characteristic. It is possible to possess any one of the following physical fitness aspects in varying degrees: cardiovascular fitness, muscular endurance, strength, body composition, power, speed, agility, balance, coordination, reaction time, and flexibility.

3. *Cardiovascular fitness, muscular endurance, strength, body composition, and flexibility may be considered the health-related aspects of physical fitness,* (62)

4. The health-related fitness aspects as listed above can contribute to a state of positive health by reducing chances of degenerative diseases, increasing work efficiency, and eliminating muscle soreness.

5. *Power, speed, agility, coordination, balance, and reaction time contribute to one's ability to perform skills and to participate in enjoyable leisure-time activities.* (62)

   These aspects of physical fitness are considered as being motor or skill-related.

6. *Physical fitness needs depend upon the individual.* p3

   Several generations ago Americans performed vigorous physical activity as a way of life. More recently the need for physical exertion as part of one's job has decreased. For this reason, many individuals feel little need for physical fitness for efficient daily work. While it is true that an individual's occupation will affect his need for physical fitness, it is not true that there is little need for physical fitness for those employed in sedentary occupations. *Every individual* has a need for fitness for living. The following factors should be considered.

1. Every individual should possess enough physical fitness to meet the needs of his occupation and regular daily activities.
2. In addition to normal daily physical fitness requirements, every individual should possess enough physical fitness to be capable of meeting emergency situations.
3. Finally, the individual should possess enough physical fitness to enjoy leisure-time activities at the end of a normal workday.

Physical fitness is the basis for dynamic and creative activity.

"The relationship between the soundness of the body and the activity of the mind is subtle and complex. Much is not yet understood, but we know what the Greeks knew: that intelligence and skill can only function at the peak of their capacity when the body is healthy and strong and that hardy spirits and tough minds usually inhabit sound bodies. In this sense, physical fitness is the basis of all activities in our society; if our bodies grow soft and inactive, if we fail to encourage physical development and prowess, we will undermine our capacity for thought, for work, and for the use of those skills vital to an expanding and complex America." (145)

Suggested Readings

Cooper, K. H. *The New Aerobics.* New York: M. Evans Co., 1970.
——— and Cooper, M. *Aerobics for Women.* New York: M. Evans Co., 1972.
The Physical Fitness Research Digest. Published quarterly by the President's Council on Physical Fitness and Sport. Available in most libraries.

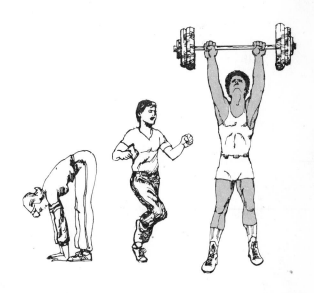

Cardiovascular fitness, muscular endurance, strength, body composition, and flexibility are health-related aspects of physical fitness.

Health-Related Fitness

Concept 3

Cardiovascular fitness, muscular endurance, strength, body composition, and flexibility are health-related aspects of physical fitness.

Introduction

As previously indicated, physical fitness consists of at least eleven specific aspects. An individual might perform well in one area without performing well in others. All aspects of physical fitness are important; however the aspects of cardiovascular fitness, muscular endurance, strength, body composition, and flexibility are most important to good health. An individual must possess more than minimal amounts of these fitness aspects if "hypokinetic diseases" are to be prevented.

Terms

Threshold of Training—The intensity, frequency, and duration of exercise necessary to cause an improvement in a specific aspect of physical fitness.

The Overload Principle—A basic principle of physical activity that indicates that for an aspect of fitness to improve one must "overload" or do more than normal exercise relating to that aspect of fitness.

The Facts

Benefits

Persons who possess cardiovascular fitness have less risk of coronary heart disease and other hypokinetic diseases. (102, 74, 202, 211)

Persons who possess good muscular endurance and strength have greater working capacity, less chance of injury, and less risk of contracting hypokinetic diseases, such as low back pain. (164, 167, 97)

Persons who possess good flexibility are less likely to injure muscles and

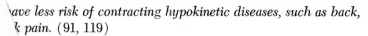

ave less risk of contracting hypokinetic diseases, such as back,
k pain. (91, 119)

body composition consisting of high amounts of lean muscle
se and other health problems than those who are overfat.

There is evidence that those people who are too fat have a higher death
rate than lean people. Among the diseases more common to obese people
are coronary heart disease, hypertension, and diabetes.

The overload principle is the basis for improving the health-related as-
pects of physical fitness. (63, 45)

In order for a muscle (including the heart muscle) to get stronger, it must
work against a greater than normal load. To increase flexibility, a muscle
must be stretched beyond its normal length. To increase muscular endurance, muscles must be exposed to sustained work. If a muscle is used
less than normal, it will atrophy, resulting in loss of strength, endurance
and flexibility.

There is no substitute for overload in developing health-related fitness.
(63, 45)

During childhood and adolescence the health-related fitness aspects may
be developed through the vigorous play activities of youth. The more
sedentary adult must make a special effort to find activities that overload the muscles and cardiovascular system.

All individuals can gain health-related fitness as a result of regular vig-
orous exercise.

Regardless of age, sex, or even current fitness status, progressive overload can benefit almost all individuals. It does not take skill in sports and
games to become fit. There are cardiovascular fitness, strength, muscular
endurance, and flexibility exercises, as well as exercises for reducing body
fatness, which are appropriate for *all* individuals. Even those who have
previously experienced heart attacks can benefit from regular progressive
exercise. (206)

Overload should be progressive. (63, 45)

Exercises should be specifically selected to meet specific purposes. There
is an optimal amount of exercise for building health-related fitness. Too
little exercise may be no more valuable than no exercise at all. Too much
exercise may be less valuable than no exercise at all and can be dangerous.

To work within the "threshold of training" is an example of progressive overload.

There is a "threshold of training" that is unique to each aspect of health-related fitness.

"Threshold of training" refers to the amount of exercise that should be done to produce fitness gains. To work above or below the threshold of training is ineffective. The threshold of training for each of the health-related fitness aspects will be described in the following chapters.

The "threshold of training" includes three different variables that must be considered when exercising to improve health-related physical fitness.

1. Intensity. Exercise must be hard enough to require more exertion than normal.
2. Duration. Exercise must be done for a significant length of time to be effective. As duration increases, intensity may be decreased.
3. Frequency. Exercise must be performed regularly to be effective. Even exercise of enough intensity and duration may not be effective in improving health-related fitness if not performed regularly.

Suggested Readings

American College of Sports Medicine. *Encyclopedia of Sports Science and Medicine.* New York: Macmillan, 1971, pp. 280, 1067-68, 1078, 1160, 1338-40.
President's Council on Physical Fitness and Sports. "Effects of Chronic Exercise on Cardiovascular Function." In *Physical Fitness Research Digest,* July 1972.
———. "Development of Muscular Strength and Endurance." In *Physical Fitness Research Digest,* January 1974.
———. "Joint and Body Range of Movement." In *Physical Fitness Research Digest,* October 1975.

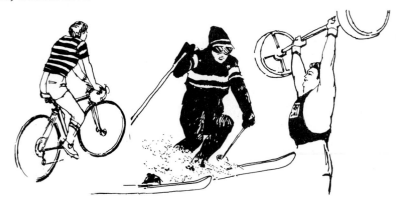

Cardiovascular fitness, the ability of the blood, heart, lungs, and other systems of the body to effectively persist in effort, is probably the most important aspect of physical fitness and can be developed and assessed in many different ways.

Cardiovascular Fitness

4

Concept 4

Cardiovascular fitness, the ability of the blood, heart, lungs, and other systems of the body to effectively persist in effort, is probably the most important aspect of physical fitness and can be developed and assessed in many different ways.

Introduction

Cardiovascular fitness is frequently considered the most important aspect of physical fitness because those who possess it are likely to have a lessened risk of coronary heart disease. Cardiovascular fitness is also referred to as cardiovascular endurance, cardiorespiratory capacity, and circulatory fitness. Whatever the word used to describe this important aspect of physical fitness, it is complex because good cardiovascular fitness requires fitness of many different body systems.

Terms

Aerobic Exercise—Exercise for which the body is able to supply adequate oxygen to sustain performance for long periods of time.

Anaerobic Exercise—Exercise that requires the use of the body's high energy fuel. This type of exercise is of short duration and does not depend on the body's ability to supply oxygen.

Continuous Exercise (aerobic exercise)—Exercise that is maintained at a fairly constant intensity for the entire exercise period.

Hemoglobin—Oxygen-carrying pigment of the red blood cells.

Intermittent Exercise (anaerobic exercise)—Relatively taxing exercise that is alternated regularly with periods of rest or mild exercise.

Liter—A metric measure of volume slightly larger than one quart.

Maximal Oxygen Uptake—A laboratory measure of fitness commonly held to be the best measure of cardiovascular fitness.

The Facts

Because of its importance to a healthy life, cardiovascular fitness is one of the most important aspects of physical fitness.

Considerable evidence exists to indicate that people who exercise regularly have a lower incidence of heart disease (74, 202, 23) and that exercise is one type of effective prescription for those who have already suffered heart attacks. (206, 250, 153)

Good cardiovascular fitness requires a fit heart muscle.

The heart is a muscle; to become stronger it must be exercised just as any other muscle in the body. If the heart is exercised regularly its strength increases, if not it becomes weaker. Contrary to the belief that strenuous work harms the heart, research has found no evidence that regular progressive exercise is bad for the normal heart. (148) In fact, the heart muscle will increase in size and power when called upon to extend itself. The increase in size and power allows the heart to pump a greater volume of blood with fewer strokes per minute. For example, the average individual has a resting heart rate between seventy and eighty beats per minute, while in a trained athlete it is not uncommon for the pulse to be in the low fifties or even in the forties.

The healthy heart is efficient in the work that it does.

The fit heart can convert about half of its fuel into energy. An automobile engine in good running condition converts about one-fourth of its fuel into energy. By comparison, the heart is an efficient machine. (197)

The heart of a normal individual beats reflexively about 40 million times a year. During this time, over 4,000 gallons (197) or 10 tons of blood (268) are circulated each day, and every night the heart accomplishes a workload equivalent to carrying a thirty-pound pack to the top of the 102-story Empire State Building. (268)

Good cardiovascular fitness requires a fit vascular system.

Blood flows in a sequence of arteries to capillaries to veins and back to the heart. Arteries always carry blood away from the heart. Healthy arteries are elastic, free of obstruction, and expand to permit the flow of blood. Muscle layers line the arteries and on impulse from nerve fibers control the size of the arterial opening. Unfit arteries may have a reduced internal diameter (atherosclerosis) because of deposits on the interior or may have hardened, nonelastic walls (arteriosclerosis).

Fit coronary arteries are especially important to good health. The blood in the four chambers of the heart does not directly nourish the heart.

Rather, numerous small arteries within the heart muscle provide for coronary circulation. Poor coronary circulation precipitated by unhealthy arteries can be the cause of a heart attack.

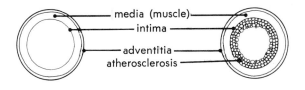

A Healthy Elastic Artery   An Unhealthy Artery

Veins have thinner, less elastic walls than arteries and contain small valves to prevent the backward flow of blood. Skeletal muscles assist the return of blood to the heart. The veins are intertwined in the muscle, and when contraction of the muscle occurs, the vein is squeezed pushing the blood on its way back to the heart. A malfunction of the valves results in a failure of used blood to be removed at the proper rate. As a result venous blood pools in the legs causing a condition known as varicose veins.

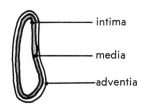

A Healthy Nonelastic Vein

Capillaries are the transfer stations where oxygen and fuel are given off to the tissues and waste products are removed from the tissues. The veins receive the blood from the capillaries for the return trip to the heart.

Good cardiovascular fitness requires a fit respiratory system, fit blood, and fit muscles capable of using oxygen. (78)

In order for a healthy heart to transmit oxygen through a healthy artery, the blood must also be healthy. It must contain adequate hemoglobin in the red blood cells (erythrocytes). Lack of oxygen-carrying capacity of the blood is called anemia.

As fit blood travels through the lungs, adequate oxygen must be transmitted from the lungs to the blood. A limited respiratory system will limit cardiovascular fitness.

If cardiovascular fitness is to be developed, one must exercise regularly within the cardiovascular threshold of training.

Research shows that three factors must be considered in designing exercise programs for developing cardiovascular fitness: frequency, intensity, and duration. (149, 216, 106, 94)

There is a threshold of training for each of two different types of cardiovascular training. (9, 149, 216)

Specific amounts of exercise necessary to achieve increases in cardiovascular fitness are outlined in Table 4.1.

Cardiovascular fitness can be achieved by doing either Aerobic or Anaerobic Exercise.

Both Aerobic (continuous) and Anaerobic (intermittent) exercise are effective in promoting cardiovascular fitness. Cooper (58) and others advocate the CONTINUOUS type program, while Astrand (9) and others recommend the INTERMITTENT type program. Table 4.2 summarizes the strengths and weaknesses of each.

Though cardiovascular fitness can be measured in many ways, maximal oxygen uptake is the best method for its evaluation. (78)

A person's maximal oxygen uptake is determined in a laboratory by measuring how much oxygen one can use in one minute of maximal work. Great endurance athletes can extract five or six liters of oxygen per minute from the environment during an all-out treadmill run or bicycle ride, as opposed to the average person who can extract only two or three liters. In order to extract a large amount of oxygen during maximal work a person must have a fit heart muscle capable of pumping large amounts of blood; fit blood capable of carrying adequate amounts of O_2; fit arteries, free from congestion and capable of carrying large amounts of blood; and fit muscles, capable of using the oxygen supplied to the muscle. Less sophisticated tests such as the twelve-minute run, the step test, or the Astrand-Ryhming Bicycle Test may also be used to measure cardiovascular endurance (see Labs 5, 6, and 7).

There is evidence that the heart should be "warmed up" before moderate to vigorous exercise. (12)

Recent research suggests (especially for middle-aged adults) the need for an adequate warm up before vigorous activity to stimuate the flow of blood to the heart muscle. This exercise should be last among warm-up exercises and should be done immediately before your planned activity begins.

Before exercising, especially sudden stopping and starting exercise like handball and basketball, you should jog easily for at least *two to three minutes*.

Table 4.1 Cardiovascular Threshold of Training*

	Continuous Exercise	Intermittent Exercise
Intensity	The heart rate should be elevated to a level as determined from your resting and maximal heart rates. (A chart is provided on page 147). Generally the heart rate should be held at a level of 135-160 beats per minute.	Short Interval Exercise: Maximal speed running, swimming, or other exercise for short distances. Rest with walking or mild exercise until the heart rate returns to 120 beats per min. Repeat as desired. Longer Interval Exercise: Exercise at 80 percent of maximum running, swimming, or other exercise speed for three to five minutes. Walk or perform mild exercise for the same length of time.
Duration	Recommended thirty minutes: Minimum: ten to fifteen minutes. As intensity increases, length of exercise periods may decrease.	Recommended thirty minutes. Minimum: ten to fifteen minutes.
Frequency	Recommended: Daily. Minimum: three times a week.	Recommended: Daily. Minimum: Three times a week.

*The threshold of training values depicted in this table are for typical adults and would need to be modified for individuals of exceptionally low or high levels of cardiovascular endurance.

Table 4.2 Advantages of Continuous and Intermittent Fitness Programs

Continuous	Intermittent
Less intense—may be better for beginners, especially those who are older and are beginning exercise after a long lay off.	May be best approach for preparing for competition, especially in sports, such as track and swimming.
Not so intense as intermittent exercise and may be easier for some people to perform regularly.	Saves time—allows a person to do more work in a given period of time.
Produces Aerobic fitness or the ability to do sustained exercise.	Produces Anaerobic fitness or the ability to do exercise involving short bursts.
Less risk to middle-age people with less than very good levels of fitness.	Some feel intermittent exercise is more interesting because it provides a "change" resulting from alternate work and rest.

Suggested Readings

Astrand, P. O. and Rodahl, K. *Textbook of Work Physiology*. New York: McGraw-Hill, 1970, chapters 6, 9, 11, and 12.

deVries, H. A. *Physiology of Exercise*. Dubuque, Iowa: Wm. C. Brown Company Publishers, 1974, chapters 6 and 19.

Lamb, L. "Exercise, Heart, and Circulation—Part I." *The Health Newsletter* 1 (1973):11.

———. "Exercise, Heart, and Circulation—Part II." *The Health Newsletter* 1 (1973):12.

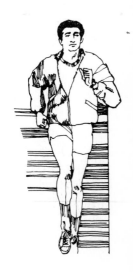

Regular exercise is one important factor in reducing the risk of coronary heart disease as well as other hypokinetic diseases.

Exercise and Heart Disease

Concept 5

Regular exercise is *one* important factor in reducing the risk of coronary heart disease as well as other hypokinetic diseases.

Introduction

There is little doubt that regular exercise is one of several important factors in reducing the risk of coronary heart disease. Statistical evidence shows "better odds" for the active individual. Presented in this unit is statistical as well as theoretical evidence relating heart disease to inactive living. Further, this unit will discuss the relationship between inactivity and other heart disease risk factors.

Terms

Angina Pectoris—Chest pain associated with lack of oxygen supply to the heart muscle.

Arteriosclerosis—A term used to describe conditions that cause the arterial walls to become thick, hard, and nonelastic; hardening of the arteries.

Atherosclerosis—A term used to describe the deposition of materials along the arterial walls; a type of arteriosclerosis.

Collateral Circulation—Development of auxiliary blood vessels that may take over normal coronary blood circulation during diminished blood flow through obstructed vessels.

Congestive Heart Failure—The inability of the heart muscle to pump the blood at a rate adequate to sustain life.

Coronary Occlusion—The blocking of the coronary blood vessels.

Coronary Thrombosis—The formation of a clot that occludes a coronary artery.

Emotional Storm—A traumatic emotional experience that is likely to affect the human organism physiologically.

Fibrin—The substance that forms a blood clot in combination with blood cells.

Hypertension—High blood pressure.

Lipid—A term used for all fats and fatty substances.

Parasympathetic Nervous System—A branch of the autonomic nervous system that slows the heart.

Risk Factor—Any of the conditions that predispose to heart disease.

Sympathetic Nervous System—A branch of the autonomic nervous system that prepares the body for activity by speeding up the heart.

The Facts

There are many different types of heart disease.

Hypertension (high blood pressure), atherosclerosis, arteriosclerosis, coronary occlusion, angina pectoris, and congestive heart failure are among the more prevalent forms of heart disease. Evidence indicates that inactivity may relate in some way to each of these types of heart disease. (24)

There is a wealth of statistical evidence that indicates that active people are less likely to have coronary heart disease than inactive people. (30, 102, 146, 118)

Much of the research relating inactivity to heart disease has come from occupational studies that show a high incidence of heart disease for persons in occupations involving only sedentary work. Even with the limitations inherent in these types of studies, the findings of more and more occupational studies present convincing evidence that the inactive individual has an increased risk of coronary heart disease. Some of the findings of more recent studies are summarized here.

1. The incidence of heart disease and coronary fatal heart attack is as much as 5.7 times greater among inactive as compared to active workers (213). While some studies only show the risk of the inactive to be two or three times greater than active people, few if any studies show no differences in heart disease between active and inactive groups.

2. There is a higher incidence of heart disease in countries with improved technology, which is related to decreasing the energy expenditure of various occupations.

3. Post-mortem studies have yielded significant information about the relationship of inactivity and heart disease. These heart examinations indicate that those involved in light work had more cardiovascular disease than those involved in heavy labor. (203)

4. Perhaps the most impressive statistics relating heart disease to inactivity come from studies of entire communities. One such study showed, in a communal society where all residents had similar diet and similar

living conditions, that inactive persons had a much higher incidence of heart disease than their active counterparts. (30) More recently, the results of a study of the residents of Framingham, Massachusetts clearly point to a lessened coronary heart disease risk for active people. (146, 74)

Contrary to popular belief, exercise does not cause "athlete's heart" nor does it injure the hearts of children. (13)

The term "athlete's heart" is a misnomer. While some investigators have found increases in heart size as a result of training, this is not the pathological increase in size associated with heart disease. There is no evidence that heavy exercise injures a normal heart.

Many parents suggest that strenuous exercise is harmful to their children. To be sure, overstrenuous activity for long periods of time may have deleterious effects, but regular activity holds no harmful effects for children's hearts. Perhaps it is the psychological and social pressures that accompany juvenile athletics that may cause unwanted results.

There are many theories that attempt to explain the causes of coronary heart disease.

Five of the most plausible theories of heart disease are the "Lipid Deposit Theory," "the Fibrin Deposit Theory," "the Coronary Collateral Circulation Theory," the "Loafer's Heart Theory," and the "Oygen Pump Theory." There is evidence that regular exercise relates in some way to each of these theories.

The Lipid Deposit Theory

There is evidence that exercise can reduce lipid deposit atherosclerosis and thus help reduce risk of heart attack. (145, 110)

The heart has its own arteries that supply blood to the heart muscle. If these vessels become clogged there is danger of a heart attack. The "Lipid Deposit Theory" of heart disease suggests that one of the causes of heart disease may be the narrowing of the artery within the heart resulting from fat or lipid deposits on the walls of these arteries (atherosclerosis). If the deposits on the inner walls of the arteries become excessive there is a diminished blood flow to the heart. Also, there is increased danger of a heart attack as a result of a clot lodging in the already narrowed coronary artery (coronary thrombosis).

There are many different kinds of blood fats including lipoproteins, phospholipids, triglycerides, and cholesterol. While cholesterol is the most well known, it may be no more the culprit than the other fats. What-

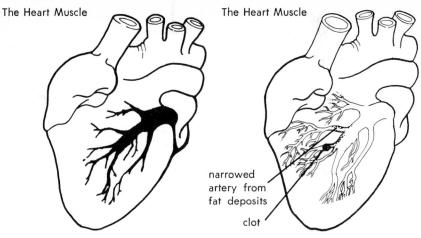

The Heart Muscle
The Heart Muscle

narrowed
artery from
fat deposits
clot

Open, Healthy Coronary Arteries
Unhealthy Coronary Arteries

ever the fat involved, the following conclusions are warranted based on recent research:

1. Exercise can reduce blood fat levels, particularly for individuals who have above normal blood fat levels. (126, 145, 102, 22)
2. There is evidence that there is an increased risk of coronary heart disease with increased blood fat levels. (146, 212, 22, 236)

The Fibrin Deposit Theory

There is evidence that regular exercise can reduce fibrin deposit atherosclerosis and thus help reduce the risk of heart attack.

Fibrin is a sticky threadlike particle that is present in the bloodstream. It is an important substance in the blood clotting process. The "Fibrin Deposit Theory" of heart disease suggests that the narrowing of the wall of the artery (atherosclerosis) may result from fibrin deposits. A heart attack may result from the diminished flow of blood to the heart resulting from the fibrin deposits or as a result of a clot lodged in the *now* narrowed artery.

The Fibrin and Lipid deposit theories are compatible, since it may be the deposit of both the sticky fibrin and fat that is responsible for atherosclerosis. If this theory is correct, exercise may help prevent a heart attack. The following research findings form the basis for this statement:

1. Exercise causes the breakdown of fibrin in the blood, thus reducing fibrin levels in the blood. (33, 186, 163)

2. Reduced blood fibrin may diminish the chances of development of fibrin atherosclerosis. (33, 186, 163)
3. Reduced blood fibrin as a result of exercise may reduce the chance of a clot forming in the blood vessel. (186, 163, 158, 273)

Coronary Collateral Circulation Theory

There is evidence that regular exercise can improve coronary collateral circulation and thus reduce the risk of a heart attack.

Within the heart there are many tiny branches of the coronary arteries that supply blood to the heart muscle. These interconnecting arteries can supply blood to any region of the heart as it is needed. "If a person is relatively inactive these interconnecting arteries are functionally closed." (173) During regular exercise these "extra blood vessels" are opened up to provide the heart muscle with the necessary blood and oxygen. For a person with atherosclerosis (and evidence suggests most of us have some atherosclerosis beginning early in life) or a person who has suffered a heart attack, coronary collateral circulation may be very important. There is also evidence that the size of the coronary arteries increases as a result of exercise. (173)

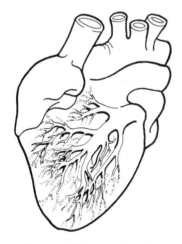 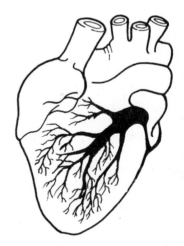

Dormant Coronary Arteries   Open Coronary Collateral Arteries

   Improved coronary circulation may provide protection against a heart attack because a larger artery would require more atherosclerosis to occlude it. In addition, the development of collateral blood vessels supplying the heart may diminish the effects of an attack if one does occur.

These "extra" (or collateral) blood vessels may take over the function of regular blood vessels during a heart attack. (87, 34, 144, 260, 118, 173)

The Loafer's Heart Theory

The heart of the inactive person is less able to resist stress and is more susceptible to "an emotional storm" that may precipitate a heart attack. (24, 167)

The heart is rendered inefficient by the following circumstances: high heart rate, high blood pressure, and excessive stimulation. Any of the above conditions require the heart to use more oxygen than normally necessary and decrease the heart's ability to adapt to stressful situations.

The "Loafer's Heart" is one that beats rapidly because it is dominated by the sympathetic nervous system, which speeds up the heart rate. Thus, the heart continually beats rapidly, even in resting situations, and never has a true rest period. Further, high blood pressure makes the heart work harder and contributes to its inefficiency. (167)

Research indicates the following concerning exercise and the "Loafer's Heart."

1. Regular exercise leads to parasympathetic dominance rather than sympathetic dominance: thus heart rate is reduced and the heart works efficiently. (24, 70, 167)
2. Regular exercise helps the heart rate return to normal faster after emotional stress.
3. Regular exercise strengthens the "Loafer's Heart" making the heart more able to weather "emotional storms." (24, 167, 222, 174)
4. Regular exercise may be one effective method of reducing high blood pressure. (25)
5. Regular exercise decreases sympathetic dominance and its associated hormonal effects on the heart, thus lessening the chances of altered heart contractibility and the likelihood of the circulatory problems that accompany this state. (222, 174)

The Oxygen Pump Theory

There is evidence that regular exercise will increase the ability of the heart muscle to pump blood as well as oxygen.

The "Oxygen Pump Theory" suggests that a fit heart muscle is one that is able to handle any "extra" demands placed on it. Through regular exercise the heart muscle gets stronger and therefore pumps more blood with each beat resulting in a lessened heart rate and a greater heart efficiency. Of importance is the fact that the heart is just like any other muscle, it must be exercised regularly if it is to stay fit.

The theories of heart disease are compatible and it is likely that most cases of coronary heart disease may be related in some way to more than one theory.

It is likely that any or all of the listed theories are correct and that exercise may help reduce the incidence of coronary heart disease in several ways. Since recent evidence indicates a decreased age for the onset of coronary heart disease, it seems especially important that we consider any factor that might reduce heart attacks. (24)

There is no single cause or prevention of coronary heart disease. However, exercise is one of several factors that significantly relates to the incidence of coronary heart disease.

Exercise may alter certain coronary risk factors and thus reduce the chances of heart disease. (24)

Certain factors or characteristics have been identified or associated with susceptibility to coronary heart disease.

While the relationship between these risk factors and coronary heart disease is of a statistically associative nature, sufficient data have been collected from a number of independent sources that suggest that physical activity may have a definite influence on several of these risk factors if not on coronary heart disease directly. See Table 5.1.

Table 5.1   Exercise and Coronary Heart Disease Risk Factors

Risk Factors	Effect of Exercise
Obesity and overfatness	Loss of fat or maintenance of weight
Excess stress and tension	Release of and increased tolerance for stress
High blood fat level	Reduction of lipid levels
Lack of exercise (activity)	Negates this factor
Age	Retards aging process
Hypertension	May reduce blood pressure for some

In addition to reducing the risk of coronary heart disease by reducing the risk factors suggested in Table 5.1, there are other benefits to the circulatory system that may result from regular exercise.

1. Regular exercise may be *one* effective method of reducing high blood pressure (hypertension). (25, 172)
2. Regular exercise is necessary for the efficient return of venous blood to the heart after it is pumped to the body parts. People in standing occupations, such as barbers, dentists, etc., can improve venous return by regular exercise, especially exercise of the leg muscles. Excessive pooling of the blood in the legs resulting from inactivity may result in varicose veins.
3. There is some evidence that regular exercise may improve peripheral circulation (circulation to the arms, legs and body parts other than the heart). (23, 46)

Exercise is only one of many factors that relates to reducing the risk of coronary heart disease.

Other major risk factors include family history of heart disease, smoking, sex, age, diet, stress, and blood pressure.

Suggested Readings

Boyer, J. M. "Effects of Chronic Exercise on Cardiovascular Function." In *Physical Fitness Research Digest,* July 1972, pp. 1-15. Available in most libraries and from the President's Council on Physical Fitness and Sports, Washington, D. C. 20201.

Fox, S. M., Naughton, J. P., and Garman, P. A. "Physical Activity and Cardiovascular Health." *Modern Concepts of Cardiovascular Disease,* Part I, April 1972, pp. 17-20.

American Heart Association Brochures. "Reduce Your Risk of Heart Attack" and "Questions and Answers about Heart and Blood Vessel Disease." Available from local Heart Association chapters.

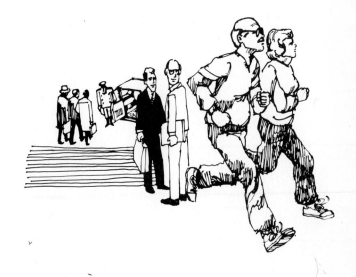

Strength and muscular endurance are two important components of physical fitness and are needed in varying degrees in all types of work and play.

Strength and Muscular Endurance

Concept 6

Strength and muscular endurance are two important components of physical fitness and are needed in varying degrees in all types of work and play.

Introduction

The development and maintenance of strength and muscular endurance is essential for a healthy life, since both strength and muscular endurance are needed to perform normal daily functions. The purpose of this concept is to clarify strength and muscular endurance terminology, present information concerning muscular contractions, and present methods of developing strength and muscular endurance.

Terms

Antagonist Muscle—The muscle or muscle group that must relax in order that movement can take place.

Concentric—An isotonic contraction in which the length of the muscle decreases.

Eccentric—An isotonic contraction in which the muscle length increases.

Isokinetic—A contraction against a controlled maximum resistance throughout the full range of motion.

Isometric—A type of muscular contraction in which the muscle's length does not change and no movement occurs.

Isotonic—A type of muscular contraction in which the muscle length changes and movement occurs.

Muscle Fiber—A single muscle cell.

Muscular Endurance—The capacity of a muscle to continue contracting over a period of time.

Repetitions—The number of consecutive times a particular movement or exercise is performed.

Set—The number of groups of repetitions of a particular movement or exercise.

Strength—A measure of the amount of external force that a muscle or group of muscles can exert.

The Facts

There are three types of muscle tissue.

The three types of muscle tissue—smooth, cardiac, and skeletal—have different structures and functions. Smooth muscle tissue consists of long spindle-shaped fibers; each fiber usually contains only one nucleus. The fibers function as the movers of internal organs since they are located in the walls of these body parts. Cardiac muscle tissue, as the name implies, is found only in the heart. Its fibers are interwoven. Smooth muscles and cardiac muscles operate involuntarily. Skeletal muscle tissues consist of long, cylindrical, multinucleated fibers. They provide the force for the movement of the skeletal system and may be controlled voluntarily.

Muscle tissue acts according to basic physiological principles. These principles may be summarized as follows:

Overload Principle—In order to promote a gain in strength, the work load for a muscle group must be greater than that to which the individual is accustomed. Contracting the muscle against a load greater than normal increases muscle strength; contracting against loads less than normal results in loss in strength and atrophy of the muscle. This same principle holds true for development of other aspects of physical fitness.

Principle of Specificity—The type and amount of strength gain is dependent upon the type and amount of exercises performed. (134) Work against near-maximum resistance with few repetitions builds muscle size and strength, while light resistance exercise with many repetitions develops muscular endurance with only slight increase in strength.

Principle of Progression—Although strength, endurance, and flexibility are developed through overload, excessive overload may cause soreness and injury rather than muscle development. Progressive overload is a gradual systematic increasing of the load over a period of time. As muscle adapts the overload should be progressively increased. Muscular endurance is developed by progressively increasing the number of repetitions of a specific task. Flexibility is progressively increased by gradually stretching the muscle farther and farther. (45, 49)

All-or-None Principle—A muscle fiber contracts completely or not at all. Theoretically, if a muscle could lift a maximum of forty pounds and was called on to lift only ten pounds then only 25 percent of the muscle fibers would contract while the other 75 percent would rest. If the muscle continued to lift the ten-pound weight the initial contracting muscle fibers would rest and additional muscle fibers would carry out the work.

Muscle Recruitment Principle—The nervous system "recruits" groups of muscle fibers according to the job to be done. If the task is slight, a few groups of fibers are stimulated; if it is heavy, many groups are recruited.

There is a proper way to perform strength and muscular endurance exercises. (187)

In utilizing different types of muscle contraction to develop strength, there are certain guidelines to which one should adhere in order to obtain maximum benefit. General guidelines for performing any type of strength exercises are summarized in Table 6.1.

Table 6.1   General Guidelines for Strength Development*

---

1. Obtain and record body measurements in order that areas needing development can be identified and progress charted.
2. Warm up slowly and completely.
3. Perform exercises at a moderate pace.
4. Select exercises for all body parts and muscle groups.
5. Perform a complete set of an exercise before proceeding to the next exercise.
6. Do not stop a workout abruptly; cool down by continuing mild exercise of the large muscles.
7. Do not expect changes overnight.

---

*Adapted from Emil Mamaliga, *Body Development Through Weight Training*. Minneapolis: Burgess Publishing Company, 1976.

The development of strength in women can be accomplished without loss of femininity.

While women need to strengthen muscles to improve their figures and develop physical fitness, there are those who prefer to avoid looking "muscular." Since some women in athletics are very muscular, some people associate strength development in women with bulging muscles. Research has shown that this association probably stems from the fact that muscular women are apt to be more successful in such sports as track and field. However, it has been shown that properly designed exercise programs actually contribute to attractive appearance, and because of a difference in hormones between males and females, there is very little likelihood that the average female will be able to develop bulging muscles. (28, 193)

Isotonic exercises are one method of effectively developing muscle strength.

Isotonics are contractions of muscles against a moveable resistance, such as barbells, weight machines, or other such equipment. This method of strength development has been used for many years.

In utilizing isotonics to develop strength, there are certain principles that should be observed in order to obtain maximum benefit. These principles are summarized in Table 6.2.

Table 6.2 Principles of Isotonic and Isometric Exercise*

Isometrics	Isotonics
1. Use maximal contractions.	1. Perform between 5 and 8 repetitions of each exercise.
2. Hold contractions 5 to 8 seconds	2. Perform three sets of each exercise. (5-8 repetions three times.)
3. Repeat several times a day.	3. During the first set lift one half maximum, during the second, three quarters, and during the third lift the maximum load.
4. Perform contractions at various joint angles.	4. Work out three to five times a week.
5. For strength in movement performance, some movement of the joint should be allowed.	5. Perform exercises for all body parts.
6. Exercise all muscle groups.	6. Work slowly, lift the weights don't throw them.

*Adapted from deVries, H. A. *Physiology of Exercise*. Dubuque, Iowa: Wm. C. Brown Company Publishers, 1974.

Research has shown that isotonic exercise will result in strength gains (15, 45, 49), however, isotonic exercises have certain advantages and disadvantages (see Table 6.3).

Specific isotonic and isometric exercises for strength development are presented in Lab 34 (Weight Training) and Lab 35 (Isometrics).

Isometric exercises are another method for developing muscular strength.

Isometrics are static muscle contractions performed against an immovable object, such as a wall, doorjamb, or against one's own antagonistic muscles. Guidelines for using isometric exercises are presented in Table 6.2.

Research has shown that isometric exercises will result in strength gains (38, 45, 49, 225, 248), however, isometric exercises have certain advantages and disadvantages (see Table 6.3).

Table 6.3 Advantages and Disadvantages of Isometric and Isotonic Exercise*

Isometrics	Isotonics
1. The major advantage is the fact that isometrics can be done in small areas without equipment.	1. Both methods build strength, but comparisons show isotonics to promote more gain.
2. One problem with this type exercise is the inability of some to be motivated to maximal performance.	2. Most work involves movement. Since isotonic exercises are movement exercises they are most likely to improve one's ability to do work.
3. Isometric contractions may impair endurance and circulatory blood flow.	3. Isotonic exercises provide some aid to endurance performances.
4. Isometrics do not build strength at all joint angles.	

*Adapted from deVries, H. A. *Physiology of Exercise.* Dubuque, Iowa: Wm. C. Brown Company Publishers, 1974.

Isometric and isotonic exercises can be combined to serve as an effective method of developing strength.

In order to incorporate the advantages of both isotonic and isometric exercise many isometric-isotonic exercises have been developed along with various machines employing the characteristics of both. Studies show that isotonic training is superior to isometric training in developing muscular strength, muscular endurance, and in recovery from muscular fatigue. (261, 262) In addition, motivation has been found to be greater in isotonic training than in isometric training. (45)

Isokinetic exercises are effective in developing muscular strength. (124, 271, 214)

A recent innovation in strength training uses slow-moving contractions done throughout a full range of movement against a constant resistance.

Machines have been developed that can be used for isokinetic exercise. Experiments show that isokinetic exercises can be effective in developing muscular strength. (124, 271, 203)

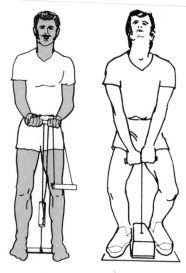

Isokinetic Exercise Devices

Concentric isotonic exercises are most effective in building strength.

It has been found that the numbers of fibers involved in muscular contractions applied to a given load differ with types of contractions used. Concentric contractions involve the greatest number of muscle fibers with isometric contractions involving the next greatest number. Eccentric contractions involve the least number of the three types of contractions. Since tension exerted by a muscle is the important factor in building strength (109), one can conclude that isotonic concentric contractions are most effective in developing strength, followed by isometric contractions and eccentric contractions. (226)

Strength aids in sports performance. (16, 43, 48, 272)

Strength development whether isometric, isotonic, or isokinetic has been shown to produce improvements in many motor performances; exercise programs designed to strengthen muscles primarily involved in a particular sport can be used as supplements to regular practice in effectively improving one's skills and motor fitness. Generally, improved strength is associated with improved speed of movement and improved muscular power.

Repetition of a muscular contraction provides the basis for development of muscular endurance. (45)

Muscular endurance is developed by progressively increasing the number of repetitions of an exercise when only light resistance is used. (17, 37, 42, 44, 248, 263) Muscular strength may also be enhanced by endurance training but to a lesser degree than with strength training.

Specificity of training is desirable if one is to expect a maximum transfer of training effect.

In the training program, one should simulate as nearly as possible the movement conditions that will be encountered in the physical activity to be performed. This simulation will help the athlete to obtain optimum results.

Strength, once gained, may persist for some time before it gradually returns to pretraining levels. (42)

It has been found that some strength has been retained for several months with the greatest loss in strength occurring during the first three or four weeks after training ceases. (42)

Suggested Readings

Mamaliga, Emil. *Body Development Through Weight Training.* Minneapolis: Burgess Publishing Co., 1976.

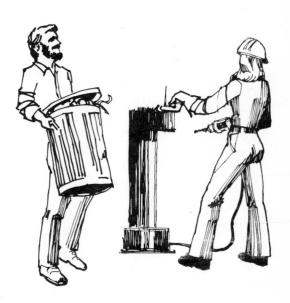

Adequate flexibility permits freedom of movement and may contribute to ease and economy of muscular effort, success in certain sports, and less susceptibility to some types of muscular injuries.

Flexibility

7

Concept 7

Adequate flexibility permits freedom of movement and may contribute to ease and economy of muscular effort, success in certain sports, and less susceptibility to some types of muscular injuries.

Introduction

Flexibility is a measure of the range of motion available at a joint or a group of joints. It is determined by the shape of the bones and cartilage involved in the joint and by the length of the ligaments and muscles that cross the joint. It is an often overlooked component of physical fitness that may become a concern of the average person only after the joints stiffen and muscles shorten from disuse, injury, or disease.

There is a wide range of flexibility possessed by different individuals. At one extreme is a significant lack of flexibility, which is evidenced by impaired and perhaps painful performance. At the other extreme is the high degree of flexibility (sometimes referred to erroneously as "double-jointedness") required for success by the acrobat, contortionist, escape artist, gymnast, and dancer. Each person, depending on individual needs, must have a reasonable amount of flexibility to perform effectively for daily living.

Terms

Ballistic Stretch (Dynamic Stretch)—Type of stretching exercise involving a bouncing or jerking motion to gain momentum in the body part in order to stretch farther.

Dysmenorrhea—Painful menstruation.

Elasticity—Property of tissue that allows it to regain its original length after being stretched.

Extensibility—Property of tissue that allows it to be stretched beyond its resting length.

Flexibility—Range of motion available in a joint or a group of joints. Mobility.

Hamstrings—Muscles that cross the back of the hip joint and the back of the knee joint, causing hip extension and knee flexion.

Ligaments—Bands of connective tissue that connect bones to bones.

Lumbar Muscles—Erector spinae and other muscles of the lower back (lumbar) region of the spine.

Reciprocal Innervation—When a muscle (agonist) contracts, its opposing muscle (antagonist) will reflexively relax.

Static Stretch—Slow, sustained stretching exercise that places a muscle in a lengthened position and holds the position for a few seconds.

Stretch Reflex—When a muscle is placed on sudden stretch, it will reflexively contract as a protective measure.

Tendons—Bands of connective tissue that attach muscles to bones.

The Facts

Flexibility is specific to each joint of the body.

No one flexibility test will give an indication of one's overall flexibility. For example, "tight hamstrings" might be revealed in a toe-touch test, but the range of motion in other joints may be quite different. (19)

Lack of use, injury, and disease may cause a decrease in joint mobility.

Arthritis and calcium deposits may damage a joint, and inflammation may cause pain that prevents movement. Failure to regularly move a joint through its full range of motion may lead to a foreshortening of muscles and ligaments; static positions held for long periods of time, such as in poor posture or when a body part is immobilized in a cast, lead to shortened tissue and loss of mobility. Improper exercise that overdevelops one muscle group while neglecting the opposing group results in an imbalance that restricts flexibility. (169, 206, 269)

The length of body parts does not significantly affect flexibility.

Contrary to popular opinion, there is no relationship between leg length or trunk length and the scores made on flexibility tests. (116, 117)

Flexibility has been found to be influenced by age and sex.

As children grow older, they increase in flexibility until adolescence when they become progressively less flexible with age. As a general rule, girls tend to be more flexible than boys. This is probably attributable to anatomical differences in the joints as well as differences in the type and extent of activities the two sexes tend to choose. (113)

Scores on flexibility tests may be affected by several factors other than joint structure.

Range of motion may vary considerably with effort, warm-up before starting the test, presence of muscle soreness and tolerance for pain, room temperature, and the individual's ability to relax. (245)

Adequate flexibility may help prevent muscle strain and orthopedic problems such as backache.

Short, tight muscles are more apt to be injured by overstretching than are long muscles. One common cause of backache is shortened lumbar and hip flexor muscles. (184, 196, 234) A further discussion of problems of the back is presented in Concept 13.

It is not necessary to sacrifice flexibility in order to develop strength.

A person with bulging muscles may be "muscle-bound" (lack of flexibility), but only if he or she trained improperly. In any progressive resistance program both agonists and antagonists should receive equal attention and all movements should be carried through the full range of motion. (29, 127)

Good flexibility may bring about improved athletic performance.

A hurdler must have good hip joint mobility to clear the hurdle. A swimmer requires shoulder and ankle flexibility for powerful strokes. A diver must be able to reach his toes in order to perform a good jacknife. Low back flexibility allows a runner to lengthen his stride. The fencer needs long hamstrings and hip adductors in order to lunge a long distance. (26, 127)

Too much flexibility in certain joints may make one more susceptible to injury.

Muscles and tendons have both extensibility and elasticity. Ligaments are extensible but lack elasticity. When stretched, ligaments remain in a lengthened state. When this occurs, the joint lacks stability and may be susceptible to chronic dislocation or movement in an undesired plane. This is particularly true of weight-bearing joints such as the knee joint. Loose ligaments may allow the knee to twist or move laterally, tearing the cartilage and damaging other soft tissue. (269)

Exactly how much flexibility an individual should possess has not as yet been scientifically demonstrated.

There are test norms available that tell us how various subjects perform on flexibility tests, but we are not certain that the old adage "the more, the better" is true. Too much flexibility may be as detrimental as too little. (189)

Flexibility may be increased (within limits) by the regular and repeated performance of static exercise or by ballistic stretching exercise.

There is a great deal of misunderstanding and controversy about static vs. ballistic stretching methods, but there appear to be advantages and disadvantages to each type of flexibility exercise. Both must use the overload principle to be effective (i.e., the muscle must be stretched beyond its normal length). (19, 77, 127, 168, 184) Table 7.1 presents a comparison of the two types of exercises.

Table 7.1 Comparison of Advantages and Disadvantages of Static vs. Ballistic Stretching Exercises

Static	Ballistic
1. Safer; less apt to overstretch the muscle or cause muscle soreness.	1. More apt to cause injury by overstretch, especially in the presence of old injury where scar tissue is present. Contraindicated in presence of pathology.
2. Requires use of a partner or outside force greater than that which can be provided by contraction of opposing muscle group.	2. Utilizes momentum to provide the overload.
3. Is probably less effective on trunk and leg flexibility.	3. Is probably more effective on trunk and leg flexibility (although some research studies find no differences).
4. Will not elicit reflex contraction (stretch reflex) of the stretched muscle.	4. Will elicit the reflex contraction, but this is not detrimental to flexibility because the muscle will not be overlooked during contraction, since momentum has been spent.
5. Does not take advantage of the reciprocal innervation that would cause the stretched muscle to relax and be capable of greater extensibility. (Note: The individual can be taught to consciously contract the opposing muscle group to facilitate the reflex relaxation.)	5. Since the opposing muscle group usually produces the movement, the muscles being stretched will relax by virtue of reciprocal innervation, permitting greater stretch.
6. Can be used to relieve some types of muscle soreness.	

There is some evidence to indicate that proprioceptive neuromuscular facilitation (PNF) techniques are useful in developing flexibility.

To use the PNF technique you first contract the muscle to be stretched. Then have a partner help you passively stretch it as you contract its antagonist. For example, to stretch the calf muscle, first contract the calf by pointing the toe. Then contract the antagonist by pulling your toes toward your shin as a partner stretches the calf by pushing your toe toward your shin. (127)

Stretching exercises are useful in preventing and remediating dysmenorrhea.

Painful menstruation of some types can be prevented or reduced by stretching the pelvic and hip joint fascia. (19)

Static muscle stretching appears to be effective in relieving muscle soreness and "shin splints."

One theory suggests that local muscular soreness may be caused by slight reflex contractions. There is some evidence that static stretch of the affected muscle may relieve these slight contractions and thus relieve the pain. Even some cases of nonpathological "shin splints" may be relieved by such exercise. (76, 79)

There is a proper way to perform flexibility exercises.

Guidelines are presented in Table 7.2.

Table 7.2 Guidelines for Performing Flexibility Exercises

1. Avoid ballistic exercises on previously injured muscles.
2. Avoid ballistic toe-touches in the presence of backaches.
3. If ballistic stretching is used, the bounces should be easy, gentle movements to avoid overstretching.
4. Static stretching should be repeated several times daily. During each repetition, the stretch should be held for a period of six to twelve seconds. (To provide overload the assistance of a partner may be helpful).
5. Exercises must be performed for each muscle group or joint in which increased flexibility is desired.
6. Exercises that do not cause a muscle to lengthen beyond normal may maintain flexibility but will not increase flexibility.
7. To increase flexibility the muscle must be "overloaded" (i.e., stretched beyond normal length).

Suggested Readings

deVries, H. *Physiology of Exercise for Physical Education and Athletics.* Dubuque, Iowa: Wm. C. Brown Company Publishers, 1974, chapter 22.

Obesity is a significant health problem that can be controlled, in most cases, with a proper balance between caloric consumption (diet) and caloric expenditure (physical activity).

Body Composition/ Weight Control

Concept 8

Obesity is a significant health problem that can be controlled, in most cases, with a proper balance between caloric consumption (diet) and caloric expenditure (physical activity).

Introduction

Appearance is probably the major reason why most people are concerned about weight control. However, proper body composition is also very important to total health and fitness. It is the purpose of the following discussion to present facts about weight control including information about diet and physical activity. Special consideration is given to the use of exercise as an effective means of maintaining ideal body weight.

Terms

Calorie—A unit of energy supplied by food; the quantity of heat necessary to raise the temperature of a kilogram of water one degree centigrade (actually a kilocalorie but usually called a calorie for weight control programs).

Caloric Balance—Consuming calories in amounts equal to the number of calories expended.

Diet—The usual food and drink for a person or animal.

M.E.T.—Amount of oxygen used per minute per kilogram of body weight by a resting person. It is commonly used as a unit of energy expenditure.

Obesity—Extreme weight, often considered as 20 to 30 percent above "normal," probably best defined as an overfat condition.

Overfat—Having too much body weight as fat: for men more than 20 to 25 percent of the total body weight as fat and 25 to 30 percent for women.

Overweight—Having weight in excess of normal. Not necessarily harmful if weight is lean body tissue.

Somatotype—Inherent body build; ectomorph (thin); mesomorph (muscular); endomorph (fat).

The Facts

"Overfatness" rather than "overweightness" is more important in determining obesity.

Individuals who are interested in controlling their weight usually consult a height-weight chart to determine "desirable" weight. Being 20 percent or more above ideal chart weight is the commonly accepted criterion of obesity. While proper chart weights are good general guidelines, it is now clear that for most people the height-weight chart is not as accurate an indication of obesity as is the percentage of body fat.

Underwater (hydrostatic) weighing and skinfold measurements now make it possible to estimate the percentage of the body weight that is comprised of fat. Some individuals who possess muscular body types have been shown to be overweight and even obese in terms of height-weight charts, yet they possess very little body fat. Since the amount of body fat, not the amount of weight, is the important factor in living a healthy life, it is wise to use "overfatness" rather than "overweightness" as the measure. (246, 47)

Obesity or "Overfatness" contributes to many degenerative diseases and health problems.

Research evidence indicates that the . . . "complications associated with obesity are far-reaching, being associated with serious organic impairments and shortened life, with psychological maladjustments, with unfortunate peer relationships (especially among children); with inefficiency of physical movement, and with ineffectiveness in motor and athletic activities. Obesity is consistently encountered as a cause of physical unfitness among boys and girls, men and women. . . ." (47) Fat people have a higher frequency of respiratory infections, a prevalence of high blood pressure and atherosclerosis, and are prone to disorders of the circulation, respiration and kidney systems. (47)

Overfatness or obesity may shorten life. (47)

Results of several investigations indicate that people who are moderately overfat have a 40 percent higher than normal risk of shortened life and more severe obesity yields a 70 percent higher than normal death rate. (47) This fact is substantially reflected in the exorbitant life insurance premiums of obese individuals.

Obesity is a problem experienced by too many Americans.

Some experts indicate that as many as 60 million or half of all of the adults in the United States are overweight. (135) Others suggest that at least one-third of adult Americans are "overfat." In addition to the problem of adult obesity, statistics indicate that as many as 10 million school children may be classified as "overfat" or obese. (135)

A balance in caloric expenditure and caloric intake is necessary for maintaining a desirable body fat content.

In order to lose a pound of body fat an individual must "expend" 3,500 calories more than one takes in. The reverse is true if one desires to gain a pound. Although dietary restrictions and regular exercise are both effective methods of regulating caloric balance, it is now clear that "quick reducing" plans are *not* effective in producing lasting fat losses. (210)

In some cases, "glandular" problems may cause an obese condition. However, these conditions are quite rare. Obesity is usually a result of an imbalance between caloric intake and output. Crash diets, spot reducing, and exercise "gimmick" machines are *not* effective in producing lasting fat loss. Weight losses in excess of one or two pounds a week are not likely to be lasting and are discouraged unless the loss results from a planned program under the close supervision of a physician. (47)

Exercise is one effective means of controlling body fat. (282)

There is little question that dieting will result, in most cases, in a loss in body weight. There is, however, another means for losing body fat, namely physical activity. Though physical activity or exercise will not result in immediate and large decreases in body fat levels, there is increasing evidence that fat loss resulting from exercise may be more lasting than fat loss from dieting. (1) Vigorous exercise can increase the resting energy expenditure (one MET) up to 13 times (13 METS). (10)

If a person exercises moderately for fifteen minutes a day (all other things being equal) a loss of more than ten pounds in a year's time may be seen. Regular walking, jogging, swimming, or any type of sustained exercise can be effective in producing losses in body fat. (47, 217) In fact, recent studies indicate that exercise combined with dietary restriction may be the *most* effective method of losing fat. One study of adult women indicated that diet alone resulted in loss of weight, but much of the weight was lean body tissue. For those dieting as well as exercising, there were similar weight losses, but there was a much greater loss in body fat. On the basis of this research it was suggested that all weight loss programs should combine lowered caloric intake with a good physical exercise program. (282)

Appetite is not necessarily increased through exercise.

The human animal was intended to be an active animal. For this reason man's "appetite thermostat" (called the appestat by some) is set as if all people are active. Those who are inactive do not have a decreased appetite. Likewise, if one is sedentary and then begins regular exercise the appetite does not necessarily increase because the "appetite thermostat" expects activity. Very vigorous activity does not necessarily cause an appetite increase that is proportional to the calories expended in the vigorous exercise. (47, 191)

Fat children may become fat adults.

Retention of "baby fat" is not a sign of good health. On the contrary, excess body fat in the early years is a health problem of considerable concern. As many as 25 percent of American school children are overfat. (141) Of these children, four of five will become too fat adults. Twenty-eight of twenty-nine teenagers who are too fat will become overfat adults. There is evidence that children who are obese may actually increase the number, as well as the size, of their fat cells thus making them predisposed to obesity in later life. (163)

Inactivity contributes to childhood obesity.

Studies of fat children show that activity restriction is more often a cause of obesity than is overeating. (61, 140) Many fat children eat less, but are considerably less active than are their nonfat peers.

"Creeping obesity" often accompanies increase in age.

Many of the "too fat Americans" are between the ages of thirty and sixty. As one grows older, changes in metabolism cause a decrease in caloric expenditure necessary to sustain life. Unless activity is increased or diet is restricted, a gain in weight will occur. Activity usually decreases while eating "habits" remain fairly constant with age. Thus, obesity creeps up on an individual. (191) To prevent "creeping obesity" it is suggested that the average person cut caloric intake 3 percent each decade after age twenty-five, so that by age sixty-five caloric intake is at least 10 percent less than at age twenty-five.

Suggested Readings

Mayer, Jean. *Overweight: Causes, Cost, and Control.* Englewood Cliffs, N. J.: Prentice-Hall (Spectrum), 1968.
President's Council on Physical Fitness and Sports. *Exercise and Weight Control.* A pamphlet available from the Council, Washington, D. C. 20201.

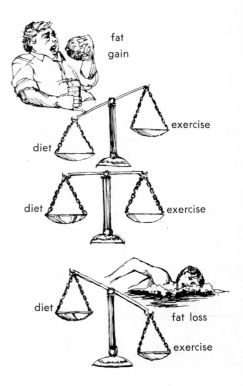

The basic nutritional needs of athletes and nonathletes do not differ except for caloric requirements. Although there are special considerations for athletes, much of their dietary practices are faddish, unsound, and even dangerous.

Exercise and Nutrition

9

Concept 9

The basic nutritional needs of athletes and nonathletes do not differ except for caloric requirements. Although there are special considerations for athletes, much of their dietary practices are faddish, unsound, and even dangerous.

Introduction

In spite of the fact that nutrition is an advanced science, many myths and misconceptions prevail. These are propagated by commercial interests that gain by the sale of their products; through ignorance of the true facts by the public and even physicians and educators; and by superstition. The latter seems to thrive particularly well among athletes and coaches. This concept will discuss some current theories and practices and attempt to dispel some myths about the feeding of athletes and people who engage in regular physical activity.

Because nutrition affects us all, it is important that we be knowledgeable about the subject. It is far too complicated to cover even the fundamentals in these pages; therefore, the reader is urged to enroll in a course on nutrition or study reliable books on the subject (see Recommended Readings at the end of this chapter), and when purchasing food, to read the nutritional label.

Terms

Cellulose—Indigestible fiber (bulk) in foods.
Kilogram—A metric unit of weight equaling 2.2046 pounds.
"Making Weight"—Quick loss or gain in weight so an athlete (usually a wrestler) can compete in a given weight category.

The Facts

The amount and kind of food one eats affects one's size, strength, and fitness.

There are about forty to forty-five nutrients contained in food that are essential for the body's growth, maintenance, and repair. These are classified into carbohydrates, fats, proteins, vitamins, minerals, and water. The first three of these provide energy, which is measured in calories.

The Food and Nutrition Board of the National Academy of Sciences—National Research Council has established "recommended daily allowances" (RDA) of the nutrients. To help assure that we select foods containing the essential elements, they have classified foods into groups, each of which should be included in the daily diet. The quantity of nutrients recommended varies with age and other considerations; for example, a young, growing child needs more calcium than an adult, and a pregnant woman needs more calcium than other women. (21)

The specified number of servings from each of the food groups on a daily basis will provide a well-balanced diet. (21)

See Table 9.1, Recommended Food Selections for Good Health, for information on the four food groups and the recommended number of daily servings.

The number of calories needed per day depends on such factors as age, sex, size, muscle mass, glandular function, emotional state, climate, and exercise.

Table 9.1 Recommended Food Selections for Good Health

Food Group	Amount for Adults	Special Role in Diet
1. Milk, cheese, ice cream, and other dairy products	2 or more servings	Protein, calcium and other minerals, vitamins
2. Meat, poultry, fish, eggs (Alternates: nuts, dried beans, peas)	2 or more servings	Protein, iron and other minerals, B vitamins
3. All vegetables and fruits, including potatoes		Minerals, vitamins, fiber
a. Green and yellow vegetables	4 or more servings	iron, vitamin A, folacin
b. Citrus fruits, tomatoes, raw cabbage, etc		vitamin C
4. Grain products—bread, flour, cereals, baked goods (preferably whole-grain or enriched)	4 or more servings	Inexpensive source of energy; iron; vitamin B

A moderately active college-aged woman needs about 2,000 calories per day, while a moderately active man of that age needs about 2,800. A female athlete in training might burn 2,600-3,500; a male athlete in training may expend 3,500-5,500. (3, 21, 190) If weight remains at the optimum, the caloric content of the diet is correct. If weight varies from optimal, then the caloric content of the diet may need to be altered.

Athletes and active people do not need relatively more protein than non-athletes or inactive people.

Protein needs vary with age, size, and other factors such as pregnancy, but the well-balanced diet includes about sixty grams of protein per day. This is well over the minimum needed and is adequate for most people. The recommended protein intake is about one gram per kilogram of body weight or 11 to 16 percent of the total calories per day.

Athletes or active people frequently consume more calories than non-athletes or inactive people; and for this reason they consume more protein, assuming that they eat a balanced diet. Because protein is not used as an important source of energy and muscular work has no effect on protein needs, there is no need to supplement the athlete or active person's diet with protein. High-quality protein is provided by all meats, milk, cheese, and eggs. Therefore, there is no reason for athletes to gorge themselves on beef steak or to take supplemental proteins if they eat a balanced diet. (3, 21, 54, 190, 192, 179)

Fat should be eaten in only moderate to low amounts.

Humans need some fat in their diet because fats are carriers of vitamins E, K, D, and A; are a source of essential linoleic acid; make food taste better; and provide a concentrated form of calories. Fat has twice the calories per gram of carbohydrates, but it does not provide twice the energy. High fat diets provide no special benefits for the active person. Most Americans consume about 40 percent of their calories in fats, but we should probably reduce this to about 25 percent to cut down on obesity and high blood fat levels in the population. (3, 21, 190)

Breakfast is an important meal.

Numerous studies have shown that omission of the breakfast meal results in poor performance because blood sugar drops in the long period between dinner the night before and lunch the following day. Persons on reducing diets probably eat more total calories when they omit breakfast because they tend to overeat at lunch and dinner. About one-fourth of the day's calories should be consumed at breakfast. (21, 190)

Some dietary practices are detrimental to performance.

Skipping meals and dehydration are two practices that are detrimental to performance. Another practice that research has shown to adversely affect performance is vitamin deficiency. A reduced intake of vitamin B and thiamin are evident within a few days. A lack of minerals has a negative effect, but it does not become evident until a few weeks (with the exception of the electrolytes [e.g., sodium and potassium, where a deficiency occurs with dehydration]). Low carbohydrate diets are also detrimental to performance. (21)

There is no scientific basis for eliminating milk from the athlete's diet.

Milk does not cause "cotton mouth." Dryness of the mouth is due to decreased saliva flow from dehydration or emotional state. Milk does *not* decrease speed, "cut wind," produce sour stomach, or interfere with performance unless the individual has an intolerance to milk. (3)

"Quick energy" foods eaten just before events of short duration do not enhance performance.

Ingesting honey, glucose, or other sweets just prior to short-term performance does not provide the athlete with a burst of energy. The body will use its own energy reserves. The carbohydrates eaten will go toward replacing the energy used in the performance. (3)

"Carbohydrate Loading" improves performance in endurance events, but it is not without hazards. (249)

Carbohydrates provide most of the energy used in heavy exercise and endurance events exceeding thirty to sixty minutes. Several studies have supported the following dietary procedures:

  a. Approximately one week before the event, exhaust the muscles to be used in the event;
  b. Four to six days before the event, eat a high protein and fat, low carbohydrate diet ("Carbohydrate Depletion");
  c. One to three days before the event, add large quantities of carbohydrates to the diet ("Carbohydrate Loading"). (3, 8, 18, 21, 179)

The "loading" procedure has been shown to improve performance for some.

One physician reports serious side effects as a result of this diet in a middle-aged marathon runner and questions its advisability for older individuals. (199) Another physician indicates that carbohydrate loading can result in cramps, increased myoglobin in the blood in amounts sufficient to result in kidney congestion, not to mention the possibility of decreased running efficiency. (249)

The timing may be more important than the makeup of the pre-event meal.

It is probably best to eat about three hours before competition to allow time for digestion. Generally the athlete can make his food selection on the basis of his past experience. Tension, anxiety, and excitement are more apt to cause gastric distress than food selection. It is generally accepted that fat intake should be minimal because it digests more slowly; "gas formers" should probably be avoided, and proteins and high cellulose foods should be kept to a minimum prior to prolonged events to avoid urinary and bowel excretion. Two or three cups of liquid (avoid caffeine) should be taken to insure adequate hydration. (3, 21) It should be noted that the excitement associated with competition is probably the main reason for having a special diet before participation.

Since many people who exercise regularly do not compete during their exercise, there is little reason to alter their normal diet before their regular exercise. Likewise, there is no need to delay exercise for long periods after the meal if exercise is to be moderate and noncompetitive.

"Health foods," tonics, and supplements will not contribute to health, fitness, weight control, or athletic performance.

The Food and Drug Administration labels the health food racket as the most widespread quackery in the United States. (254) Whether athletic or sedentary, the individual on a well-balanced diet does *not* benefit from special "organic" foods, additional vitamins (including vitamin E), choline, lecithin, wheat germ, brewer's yeast, gelatin, royal jelly, or any other supplement, unless specifically prescribed for a medical purpose by one's own physician. (3, 4, 21, 32, 190, 254)

Fad diets are not a satisfactory means to long-term weight reduction and may adversely affect the health.

There are hundreds of fad diets and diet books, but nutritionists warn that there is no scieintific basis for drastic juggling of food constituents. Such diets are usually unbalanced and may result in serious illness or even death, especially for the obese person who is already apt to be suffering from a number of health disorders. Fad diets cannot be maintained for long periods of time, therefore the individual usually regains any lost weight. Constant losing and gaining may be more harmful than the original weight condition.

Crash diets that bring about a weight loss by dehydration of only 5 percent in forty-eight hours have been shown to reduce the individual's working capacity by as much as 40 percent. The practice of "making weight" in athletics whether by dehydration, induced vomiting, or starvation diets is dangerous to health and should be condemned. (2, 3, 190, 254)

Suggested Readings

American Association for Health, Physical Education and Recreation. *Nutrition for Athletes,* 1971 (1201 16th St., N.W., Washington, D. C. 20036).

Bogert, L. J., et al. *Nutrition and Physical Fitness,* 9th edition. Philadelphia: W. B. Saunders Company, 1973.

Chicago Nutrition Association. *Nutritional References and Book Reviews,* Revised 1975 (8158 S. Kedzie Ave., Chicago, Illinois 60652).*

*This inexpensive paperback lists nutrition books by title, with brief abstracts and categorizes them under four headings:

(1) "Recommended"
(2) "Recommended for Special Purposes"
(3) "Recommended only with Reservations"
(4) "*Not* Recommended"

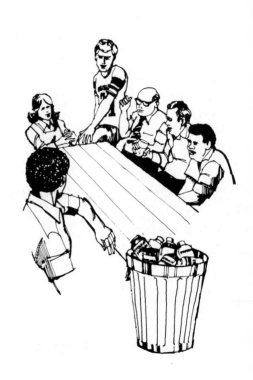

Skill-related fitness is essential to performance in games and sports as well as to working efficiency.

Skilled-Related Fitness

10

Concept 10

Skill-related fitness is essential to performance in games and sports as well as to working efficiency.

Introduction

Skill-related fitness consists of six different aspects: balance, agility, co-ordination, speed, power, and reaction time. Although these aspects of physical fitness do not necessarily make a person healthier, possession of these fitness aspects makes one better at games and sports as well as work efficiency. In a society that is becoming increasingly interested in leisure and recreation, skill-related physical fitness can be important to living a meaningful and enjoyable life.

The Facts

Good skill-related fitness may help an individual achieve good health-related fitness.

Individuals who achieve good skill-related fitness have the potential to succeed in sports and games. Regular participation in these activities can lead to improved health-related fitness throughout life. In addition, people who make an effort to learn activities involving skill-related fitness are more likely to be active in sports and games for a lifetime. (220)

Skill-related fitness may improve one's ability to work efficiently. (35)

In manual labor, skillful performance improves efficiency. For example, a ditchdigger with great ditchdigging skill uses less energy than one who has not mastered the skill. Seemingly simple skills are often quite complex and may require some proficiency in each of the skill-related fitness aspects.

Skill-related fitness may improve one's ability to meet emergency situations. (200)

Good agility would enable a person to dodge an oncoming car; good balance would lessen the likelihood of a fall; and good reaction time would decrease the chances of being hit by a flying object. Each aspect of skill-related fitness contributes in its own way to an individual's ability to avoid injury and meet emergencies.

Good skill-related fitness is beneficial to carrying out the normal daily routine and enjoying one's leisure time. (200)

Walking, sitting, climbing, pushing, pulling, and other such tasks require varying degrees of skill-related fitness. Accordingly, improvement in these aspects resulting from regular practice may improve efficiency in performing daily activities and enjoying one's leisure or recreational time.

Potential for possessing outstanding skill-related fitness is based on hereditary predispositions, but all aspects of skill-related fitness can be improved through regular practice. (242)

In order for a skill to be improved, it must be repeated. Some skill-related fitness aspects such as power, agility, balance, and coordination can be enhanced greatly with practice. Others such as speed and reaction time can be improved somewhat but are determined to a greater extent by heredity.

Exceptional athletes tend to be outstanding in more than one aspect of skill-related fitness.

While people possess skill-related fitness in varying degrees, great athletes are likely to be above average in most if not all aspects. Indeed, exceptional athletes must be exceptional in many aspects of skill-related fitness. Different sports do require different specific fitness proficiencies.

Excellence in one skill-related fitness aspect may compensate for lack of another. (231)

Each individual possesses a specific level of each of the skill-related fitness aspects. The performer should learn his strengths and weaknesses in order to produce optimal performances. For example, a tennis player may use superior shot placement to compensate for a lack of speed.

Excellence in skill-related fitness may compensate for lack of health-related fitness when playing sports and games. (267, 281)

As one grows older health-related fitness potential declines. The individual may use superior skill-related fitness to compensate. For example, a baseball pitcher who lacks the strength and muscular endurance to

Concept 10

overpower hitters may rely on knuckleball throwing skill to deceive the hitters.

Skills are specific in nature. (242)

An individual might possess ability in one area and not another. For this reason, "General Motor Ability" probably does not really exist. Individuals do not have one general capacity for performing skills. Rather, the ability to play games or sports is determined by combined abilities in each of the separate motor skill aspects of agility, coordination, balance, reaction time, speed, and power. It is, however, possible and even likely that some performers will have above-average skill in many areas.

Suggested Readings

Schmidt, R. A. *Motor Skills.* New York: Harper & Row, 1975.
Robb, M. D. *The Dynamics of Motor-Skill Acquisition.* Englewood Cliffs, N. J.: Prentice-Hall, 1972.

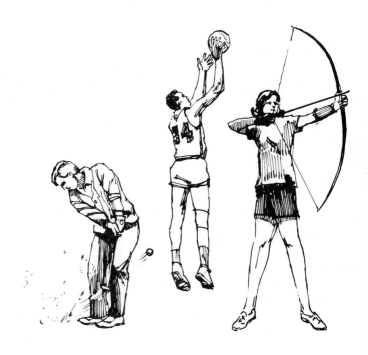

Everyone, regardless of physical abilities, can find a sport or physical activity that can be enjoyed for a lifetime.

Learning Lifetime Sports and Physical Activities

11

Concept 11

Everyone, regardless of physical abilities, can find a sport or physical activity that can be enjoyed for a lifetime.

Introduction

The recent emphasis on "lifetime sports" has seen a considerable increase in participation by American adults. However, a recent survey indicates that 45 percent or roughly 49 million American adults do not exercise on a regular basis. (220) One of the reasons for nonparticipation is that too many adults were not successful in sports activities as children. It should be emphasized that there is some type of activity that will be meaningful to every person and that lack of competitive success does not mean that a person cannot be a regular participant in exercise for a lifetime.

Terms

Lifetime Physical Activity—An activity performed after the school-age years by adults on a regular basis. These activities include those not generally considered as sports, such as walking, jogging, bicycle riding, and calisthenics.

Lifetime Sports—Sports performed after the school-age years by adults on a regular basis. Among those of greatest current popularity are bowling, swimming, golf, and tennis.

Mental Practice—Imagining the performance of a skill without actually physically performing it.

Overlearning—Practicing a skill over and over many times in an attempt to make the skill a "habit."

"Paralysis by Analysis"—Overanalysis of skill behavior. This occurs when more information is supplied than the performer can really use or when concentration on too many details of a skill results in interference with performance.

Skill Analysis—Breaking the performance of a skill into component parts and critically evaluating each phase of the performace.

The Facts

There is no one best sport or physical activity for all people.

Some people would lead us to believe that "their" sport is the "best" or "only" sport. However, while each sport has its advantages in accomplishing certain objectives, there is no single best sport for all people. The best sport or physical activity for you depends on your abilities, interests, personality, and other personal factors.

A person does not have to be a "great" performer to enjoy sports and physical activity for a lifetime.

Evidence suggests that many Americans discontinue participation in physical activity as they get older because they "are not very good at sports." There are many different types of sports and activities and each requires different abilities. Failure in the past does not mean that one cannot find enjoyment in sports in the future. Some activities require coordination, some require agility and balance, while others may require health-related physical fitness, such as cardiovascular fitness, strength, and flexibility; still others require daring or ability to use strategy. (270)

Each person should analyze his or her own personal strengths to decide which is the best activity. Some may wish to choose activities that require relatively little skill but that can be very beneficial to health and can become a meaningful part of their lifestyle. Activities such as walking, jogging, bicycle riding, and calisthenics are among the most widely used by Americans today. (220)

Participation in lifetime sports can be a means of achieving physical fitness, but it can also provide other valuable benefits as well. (156)

One of the real benefits of regular participation in lifetime physical activities can be improved health through improved cardiovascular fitness, muscular endurance, strength, and flexibility. However, the participants may also derive personal satisfaction and meaning from the participation and benefits from social interactions and the release of emotional tensions. (156)

Participation in a lifetime sport or physical activity does not insure good health-related physical fitness.

While there are many benefits to participation in lifetime physical activities, many are not of such frequency, intensity, and duration to improve health-related physical fitness. For example, in most cases bowling would do little to improve cardiovascular fitness.

While most people learn recreational sports skills early in life, lifetime sports skills can be learned at any age.

Research evidence suggests that most skills are learned early in life. In fact one study indicates that as many as 85 percent of all recreational skills are learned by the age of twelve. (205) This does not mean that "old dogs cannot learn new tricks," but it does suggest a need to teach skills to children at an early age.

Team and competitive sports provide enjoyment during our youth, but they are not activities that are likely to be engaged in as adults. (220)

A recent survey of Americans conducted by the President's Council on Physical Fitness and Sports indicated that team and competitive sports, such as football and basketball, are not as popular as activities such as swimming, bowling, golf, walking, jogging, and bicycle riding. (220)

Skill proficiency in a sport and selection of a partner of similar ability are both important to enjoyment of the sporting experience.

It is true that people who have some skill in an activity are more likely to participate in that activity than those with little or no skill. For this reason it is advisable to practice and perhaps seek instruction to enhance enjoyment of a lifetime activity. People with greater skill are more likely to get involved because they are more likely to be successful. However, there is another way to increase the satisfaction gained from sports participation. Research indicates that you must be 65 to 75 percent as good as your partner if either of you are to enjoy the activity. For this reason it is not only advisable to improve your skills, but it is suggested that you find a playing partner or group of similar ability to your own. (69)

There are certain guidelines that can be followed to help in effectively learning a lifetime sport or physical activity.

1. *When learning a new activity, concentrate on the "general idea" of the skill first; worry about details later.* For example, a diver who concentrates on pointing the toes and keeping the legs straight at the end of a "flip" may land flat on his/her back. To make it "all the way over," concentration should be on merely doing the flip. When the "general idea" is *mastered,* one can concentrate on details. (177)
2. *The beginner should be careful not to emphasize too many details at one time.* After the "general idea" of the skill is learned, then the learner begins to focus on the details, one or two at a time. Concen-

tration on too many details at one time may result in "paralysis by analysis." For example, a golfer who is told to keep the head down, to keep the left arm straight, to keep the knees bent, etc., cannot possibly concentrate on all the details at once. As a result neither the details nor the "general idea" of the golf swing are performed properly. (207)

3. *In the early stages of learning a lifetime sport or physical activity, it is not wise to engage in competition.* Research indicates that beginners who compete are likely to concentrate on "beating their opponent" rather than learning a skill properly. For example, in bowling the beginner may abandon the newly learned hook ball in favor of the sure thing" straight ball. This may make the person more successful immediately, but it is not likely to improve the person's bowling skills for the future. (276)

4. *To be performed well, lifetime sports skills must be "overlearned."* Often times when we learn a new activity, we begin to "play the game" immediately. Evidence indicates that the best way to learn a skill is to "overlearn" it or to practice it until it becomes "habit." Frequently game situations do not allow us to overlearn skills. For example, during a game is not a good time for a person to learn the tennis serve, since during a game there may be only a few opportunities to serve. For the beginner it would be much more productive to hit many serves (overlearn) with a friend until at least the "general idea" of the serve is well learned. Further, the beginner *should not* sacrifice speed to concentrate on serving for accuracy. Accuracy will come with practice of a properly performed skill. (242)

5. *Once the "general idea" of a skill is learned, an analysis of the performance may be helpful.* Being careful not to overanalyze, it may be helpful to have someone who is knowledgeable about the sport help locate strengths and weaknesses. Movies and video tapes of performances have been shown to be of help to learners. (276, 242)

6. *When "unlearning" an old (incorrect) skill and learning a new (correct) skill, performance may get worse before it gets better.* Frequently a performer hopes to unlearn a "bad habit" so as to be able to "relearn" the new or correct skill. For example, a golfer with a "baseball swing" may want to learn the correct golf swing. It is important for the learner to understand that the score may worsen during the relearning stage. As the new skill is overlearned, skill will improve, as will the golf score.

7. *Mental practice may aid skill learning.* (59, 60) Current research evidence suggests that mental practice may benefit performance of motor

skills, especially if the performer has had previous experience in performing the skill. Mental practice might be used for golf, tennis, and other sports when the performer cannot participate regularly because of the weather, business, or lack of time.

8. *For beginners, practicing in front of other people may be detrimental to learning a skill.* Research indicates that an audience may inhibit the learning of a new sports skill for the beginner. This is especially true if the learner feels that the performance is being evaluated by someone in the audience. (194)

Suggested Readings

Robb, M. D. *The Dynamics of Motor Skill Acquisition.* Englewood Cliffs, N. J.: Prentice-Hall, 1972.
Schmidt, R. A. *Motor Skills.* New York: Harper & Row, 1975.
Whiting, H. T. A. *Acquiring Ball Skill.* Philadelphia: Lea and Febiger, 1971.

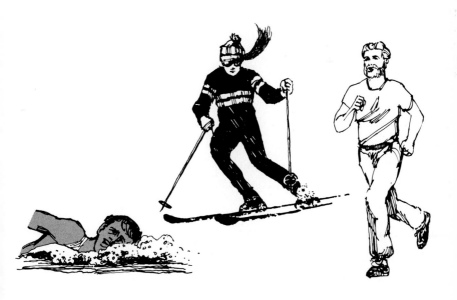

Since the human body is a system of weights and levers, its efficiency and effectiveness at rest or in motion can be improved by the application of sound mechanical and anatomical principles.

Body Mechanics

12

Concept 12

Since the human body is a system of weights and levers, its efficiency and effectiveness at rest or in motion can be improved by the application of sound mechanical and anatomical principles.

Introduction

"Body Mechanics" means the application of physical laws to the human body. The bones of the body act as levers or simple machines with the muscles supplying the force to move them. Therefore, mechanical laws may be applied to the use of the body to aid in performing more and better work with less energy while avoiding strain or injury.

In the first half of this concept, discussion is centered on the daily activities of lifting, carrying, pushing, and pulling. The last part of this concept focuses on selected mechanical principles for the fundamental techniques employed in various sport activities.

Terms

Acceleration—The rate of change of velocity.

Center of Gravity—The center of the mass of an object.

Effectiveness—The degree to which the purpose is accomplished.

Efficiency—The relationship of the amount of energy used to the amount of work accomplished.

Linear Motion—Movement in a straight line.

Locomotor movement—Movement from one place to another (i.e., running, walking, skipping).

Rotary Motion—Movement in an arc or circle around a center of rotation.

Stability—Degree of equilibrium; state of rest.

Velocity—Speed; rate of change of position.

Body Mechanics for Daily Living

The Facts About Lifting and Carrying

The best method for lifting or carrying a given object depends upon its size, weight, shape, and position in space; however, there are some general principles that should be applicable in all situations. (27, 181, 227, 274)

1. *Stand close to the object and assume a wide base.* (227, 274) Stand in a forward-backward stride position with the object at the side of the body, or assume a side-stride position with the object between the knees. The purpose of lifting from this position is that it allows one to lift straight upward from a stable position, utilizing the most efficient leverage.

2. *Keep the back straight and bend at the hips and knees. Squat, do not bend, regardless of how light the object may be.* The back was never meant to be used as a lever for lifting. Orthopedists constantly caution us against leaning forward to pick up objects without bending the knees because of the strain placed on the muscles and joints of the spine. This kind of back strain can occur when making a bed improperly or when lifting a child out of a crib. When one bends from the waist, the center of gravity of the body is higher than when one squats, thus the bending posture is less stable as well as more injurious than the squatting position.

3. *Lower your body only as far as is necessary, directly downward, keeping the hips tucked.* Squatting lower than is necessary is a waste of energy, but more importantly perhaps, deep knee bends can be damaging to the structures of the knee joints. The deeper the flexion, the greater the twist on the joint and the greater the tension in the leg muscles. (160)

4. *Grasp the object and lift with your leg muscles, keeping the object close to the center of gravity of the body.* The leg muscles are the strongest in the body, and if the back is kept erect, use of the legs for lifting allows a maximal force to be applied to the load, without wasting energy.

5. *Push or pull heavy objects if this can be done efficiently, rather than lifting.* Theoretically, it takes about thirty-four times more force to lift than to slide an object across the floor. The size, shape, and friction of the object would determine whether or not it is feasible to push or pull it. (274)

6. *Carry the object close to the body's center of gravity and no higher than waist level (except when carrying on the shoulder, head, or*

back). When objects are carried in front of the body above the level of the waist, one must lean backward to balance the load, producing an undesirable arch in the lower back. Carrying loads at the midline of the body such as in a knapsack or on the head or shoulders is effective in reducing the stress on the skeletal system. (111)

7. *Divide the load if possible, carrying half in each arm. If the load cannot be divided, alternate the load from one side of the body to the other.* When the weight is carried on one side of the body, the force on the opposite hip during walking is much greater than when the load is distributed on both sides. This is true even when the bilateral load is twice as great as the unilateral load. (278) If the weight must be carried on only one side, the opposite arm should be raised to counterbalance the load and help keep the center of gravity over the base.

8. *Avoid arching the back when lifting and lowering an object from overhead. Any lift above waist level is inefficient.* (41) Occaisonally, one must reach overhead to lift an object from a high shelf. To avoid back strain, climb a ladder or stand on a stool to prevent the necessity of raising the arms overhead. If this is not practical, reach for the object with your weight on the forward foot, then step backward on the rear foot as the object is lowered.

9. *Do not try to lift or carry burdens too heavy for you.* The most economical load for both men and women is about thirty-five percent of the body weight. Obviously, with strength training, one can safely lift a greater load.

Suggested Maximum Lifts for Persons of Average Strength (111)

	Occasional Lifts	Frequent or Continuous Lifts
Men	50 kg or 110 lbs.	18 kg or 39.6 lbs.
Women	20 kg or 44 lbs.	12 kg or 26.4 lbs.
Boys	20 kg or 44 lbs.	15 kg or 33 lbs.
Girls	11-16 kg or 24-35 lbs.	7-11 kg or 15-24 lbs.

The Facts About Pushing and Pulling

There is a controversy over whether pushing or pulling is easier; apparently it depends upon the nature of the task.

One must consider such factors as desired direction, type of movement, distance to be moved, and friction. If a downward force is desired, pushing would be best. If an upward force is desirable, pulling is probably better. Pushing tends to increase friction because of the downward force, but may offer better control since the object is closer to the person. (27, 170, 227)

Pushing and pulling are forms of lifting, therefore, the same mechanical principles may be applied.

When pushing or pulling, the back should be kept as straight as possible, a wide stance should be used, and the leg muscles should do the work rather than the back or arms. You may alternate the working muscles by changing positions occasionally, that is, face forward, then backward, then sideward. (181)

Force should be applied as nearly as possible in the desired line of direction.

If a linear motion is desired, you should apply the force at the center of gravity of the object and push or pull in the desired direction by leaning from the hips, in that direction. To move an object horizontally, the upward and downward components of the push or pull should be reduced to a minimum. When pulling, increasing the length of the handle reduces the vertical component.

If there is a great deal of friction, the force should be applied below the object's center of gravity. Sufficient force should be applied continuously to keep the load moving, since it takes more force to start an object moving (overcoming inertia) than to keep it moving. (227, 274)

When a rotary motion is desired, apply the force away from the center of gravity of the object.

Objects that are too heavy or too awkward to be moved as a whole, such as a refrigerator or couch, can be moved by applying force alternately at one end and then the other so that a pivoting or "walking" action is employed to rotate the object. (227, 274)

The Facts About Saving Energy During Work

When working with the arms in front of the body, a pulling motion is easier than a pushing motion because pulling uses the stronger flexor muscles of the arms.

To conserve energy and do a more effective job, try these suggestions. (170)

1. Painting—Paint only a foot square at a time, pushing the brush lightly, but pulling it vigorously.
2. Window washing and dishwashing—Use a counterclockwise motion

(if you are right-handed), since this puts the emphasis on the pull. It is more efficient and effective than up and down strokes.

3. Floor cleaning—In mopping, washing, and vacuuming put the pressure on the pull. The push takes twenty times more energy.
4. Ironing—Be sure the board is low enough and on a firm wide base; put the emphasis on the pull rather than the push to do a better job of ironing with less neck and shoulder strain.
5. Bedmaking—Tuck the sheet in one side, walk around the bed and pull the sheet toward you. This is thirty times more efficient than pushing out the wrinkles.

Organize work to avoid stooping or unnatural positions. (111)

1. Sideward flexion of the trunk is more strenuous than forward trunk flexion.
2. Avoid constant arm extension whether forward or sideward.
3. Try to sit while working but change to standing occasionally.
4. The arms should move either together or in opposite directions.
5. Tools most often used should be the closest to reach.
6. When working with the hands, the work bench (or kitchen cabinet) should be about 5-10 cm (2-4 inches) below the waist. The office desk should be about 74-78 cm (29-30 inches) high for the average man and about 70-74 cm (27-29 inches) high for the average woman.

Some types of arm movements are more accurate than others. (111)

Horizontal movements are more precise than vertical ones. Circular movements are better than zigzag ones. Movements toward the body are easier to control than those away from the body. Rhythmic movements are more accurate and less tiring than abrupt movements.

There is an optimum way to use tools. (111)

Shoveling—The best handle length is about 60-65 cm (23-25 inches). The best rate is twelve to fifteen shovelings per minute.
Sawing—For a two-man forest saw, the most efficient rate is forty-two double pulls per minute.
Hoeing—A swivel hoe is more efficient in soft soil. The grubbing hoe is best for hard soil.

Body Mechanics in Sports

The principles of body mechanics are the same for sports as for daily living. However, sports often require movements other than lifting, pushing, pulling, etc. For this reason selected principles of body mechanics are presented with specific attention given to efficient sports participation.

The Facts About Running and Other Locomotor Movements

There are many different ways to get from one place to another. Regardless of the locomotor movement used, whether it be running in football, the shufflestep in boxing, or backward running as in defensive basketball, there are some general guidelines that apply to most sports situations.

1. To start quickly, lean in the direction of the anticipated movement. (85, 265)
2. To stop quickly, lower the center of gravity by bending the legs, widen the base by spreading the feet and lean in the direction opposite the movement. (265)
3. To move as fast as possible, do *not* leave the ground more than necessary. The force necessary to move fast is provided by the feet or body part touching the ground. If the feet are off the ground they cannot push the body forward. (In swimming, if the hands or feet are out of the water, they cannot move the body forward). (198)
4. When moving in a circle or around a curve, centrifugal force can be counteracted by leaning into the curve, by slowing down, or by increasing the radius of the circle. (31, 139, 274)

The Facts About Jumping and/or Moving the Body in Space

Whether it be performing the long jump, the front sommersault in diving, or a gymnastics maneuver there are some basic guidelines for moving the entire body through space.

1. Once a person leaves the ground the path of the center of gravity cannot be changed. Distance cannot be added to a jump by twisting or moving the arms or legs. However, the position of the body around the center of gravity can be changed for more stability and a better landing by changing the position of the arms and legs in space. (139, 208, 274)
2. When a person is unsupported in the air, if the head moves down, the feet move up. The reverse is also true. For example, in diving, if the head goes down, the feet go up. (86, 120, 122)
3. When a person is unsupported in the air, if the head and feet move down, the hips move up. The reverse is also true. For example, the

pole vaulter lowers the head and feet to get the hips over the crossbar. (86, 120, 122)

4. The height or distance of a jump is determined by the force and velocity of movement at the moment the body leaves the ground. Optimal force can be provided for maximal vertical distance by pushing from as deep a crouch as the muscles will allow. Optimal velocity can be provided for maximal horizontal distance by having the greatest possible running speed just before the jump. (122, 224)

5. Maximal jumping distance can be obtained by transferring momentum from body parts to the total body just before leaving the ground. For example, a swimmer can reach farther at the start by thrusting the arms forward before pushing off the starting block. (218, 265)

6. When a fast turning motion of the body is required in space as in the forward somersault on the trampoline, the radius of rotation should be shortened. For example, in the somersault the legs and arms should be tucked. Conversely, to slow the turning motion of the body, lengthen the radius of rotation. An ice skater extends the arms to slow the turning motion of the body, for example. (72, 82, 83, 215, 274)

The Facts About Throwing an Object

There are some basic guidelines that should be considered for efficient throwing. Some of these guidelines also apply to jumping.

1. For maximal distance, an object such as a ball should be thrown at an angle of 45°. Because some objects tend to sail they should be thrown at a lesser angle. For example, a discus should be thrown at about 40°. A long jumper is much like a thrown ball and in theory the jump should be as near 45° as possible. However, in reality outstanding jumpers obtain the best distances at about 20°. (84, 31, 121, 198, 208, 265, 197, 250)

2. To impart as much force as possible to a thrown object, the length of the lever throwing the ball should be as long as possible when the object is released. For example, in an underhand throw, the arm should be extended at the point of release. (20, 227, 233, 274)

3. To impart as much force as possible to a thrown object, the large muscles of the body should start the movement with the smaller muscles to be added later. For example, in throwing, the legs and hips move first. When they are moving as fast as possible the upper body and arm are added. The forearm and hand are added only after the upper arm has reached its maximal velocity. (274)

The Facts About Catching or Receiving a Blow

Catching is basically receiving a blow from a thrown object. The following guidelines apply to catching a thrown object or receiving a blow of another type.

1. To avoid injury a blow should be distributed over as large an area as possible. It hurts less to catch a ball caught on all fingers than to catch a ball on one finger. A fall caught on the elbow hurts more than one on the entire arm. (31, 274)
2. When catching or receiving a ball hit off a wall, it will rebound at an angle equal but opposite the angle it hit the wall (if it is not spinning). This applies to a baseball hit off a wall, a basketball hitting the backboard, or a tennis ball hit off a rebound wall. (27, 31)

Suggested Readings

Bunn, W. *Scientific Principles of Coaching.* Englewood Cliffs, N. J.: Prentice-Hall, Inc., 1972.

Rasch, P. J. and Burke, R. K. *Kinesiology and Applied Anatomy,* 4th ed., Philadelphia, Lea and Febiger, 1971, chap. 23.

Wells, K. and Lutgens, K. *Kinesiology,* 6th ed., Philadelphia: W. B. Saunders Co., 1976.

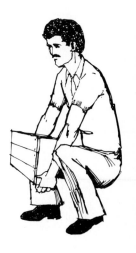

Good posture and sound care of the back can have positive effects on appearance, efficiency, effectiveness, and health.

Posture and Care of the Back

13

Concept 13

Good posture and sound care of the back can have positive effects on appearance, efficiency, effectiveness, and health.

Introduction

Good posture is something many Americans take for granted. Unless a posture problem is so severe that it affects appearance or causes pain, it may be overlooked. Likewise, care of the back often is taken for granted until some type of problem presents itself.

When considering good posture and care of the back the reader would do well to consider that early attention to good posture and care of the back can prevent problems later in life. Likewise, the reader should consider the fact that if a person already has a posture or back problem, other related problems may begin to present themselves.

Terms

Head Forward—The head is thrust forward in front of the gravity line; also called "poke neck."

Herniated Disc—The soft nucleus of the spinal disc protrudes through a small tear in the surrounding tissue; also called prolapse.

Hyperextended Knees—The knees are thrust backward in a locked position.

Kyphosis—Increased curvature (flexion) in the upper back; also called "hump back."

Lumbar Lordosis—Increased curvature (hyperextension) in the lower back (lumbar region) with a forward pelvic tilt; commonly known as "sway back."

Posture—The relationship of body parts, whether standing, lying, sitting, or moving. "Good posture" is a relationship of body parts that allows one to function most effectively, with the least expenditure of energy and with a minimum amount of strain on muscles, tendons, ligaments, and joints.

Referred Pain—A pain that appears to be located in one area while in reality, it originates in another area.

Round Shoulders—The tips of the shoulders are drawn forward in front of the gravity line.

Ruptured Disc—Spinal disc crushed from severe blow or jolt.

Sciatica—Pain radiating down the sciatic nerve in the back of the hip and leg.

Scoliosis—A lateral curvature with some rotation of the spine; the most serious and deforming of all postural deviations.

The Facts

Clinical evidence cited by physicians and educators indicate that poor posture can cause a number of health problems. For example:

1. Hyperextended knees are believed to retard blood circulation. (129)
2. Protruding abdomen and lumbar lordosis may contribute to poor circulation, painful menstruation, ruptured discs, and backache. (154, 196)
3. Forward head can result in headache, dizziness, and neck, shoulder, and arm pain. (133, 277)
4. Rounded shoulders may cause back and neck strain. (185)
5. Some postural faults cause a predisposition to certain athletic injuries. (185)
6. Imbalanced postural lines can cause neuritis, arthritis, sciatica, generalized fatigue, joint strain, and pain in the head, neck, back, hips, legs, and feet. (92, 143, 196)
7. In the presence of poor posture, organs are not given proper support and their function suffers. Posture problems relating to the chest may affect functioning of the heart and lungs in cases of disease. (154)

Good posture has aesthetic benefits.

The first impression one makes on another person is usually a visual one. Good posture can help convey an impression of alertness, confidence, and attractiveness. (181)

There is probably no one best posture for all individuals, since body build affects the balance of body parts, but in general, certain relationships are desirable. (7)

In the standing position, the head should be centered over the trunk, the shoulders should be down and back, but relaxed, with the chest high and the abdomen flat. The spine should have gentle curves when viewed from the side, but should be straight as seen from the back. When the pelvis is tilted properly, the pubis falls directly underneath the lower tip of the sternum. The knees should be relaxed, with the kneecaps pointed straight ahead. The feet should point straight ahead and the weight should be borne over the heel, the outside border of the sole, and across the ball of the foot and toes (see figure below).

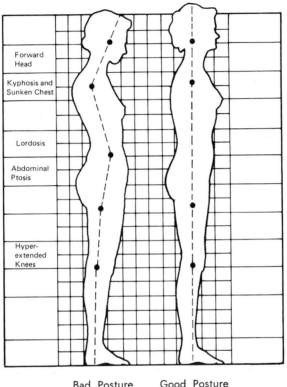

Bad Posture   Good Posture

If one part is out of line, other parts must move out of line to balance it, increasing the strain on muscles, ligaments, and joints.

The body is made in segments that are held balanced in a vertical column by muscles and ligaments. If gravity or a short muscle pulls one segment out of line, other portions of the body will move out of alignment to compensate, producing worse posture, more stress and strain, and possibly deformity in the musculoskeletal system. (196, 239)

There are many causes of poor posture, including hereditary, congenital and disease conditions, as well as certain environmental factors.

Some acquired causes of poor posture are ill-fitting clothing, chronic fatigue, improperly fitting furniture, including poor beds and mattresses; psychological problems; poor work habits; lack of physical fitness due to inactivity; and lack of knowledge regarding what constitutes good posture. (7, 92, 154, 185, 196, 224)

Approximately 80 percent of the adult population suffer from acquired foot defects. (275)

Most foot defects are acquired and are preventable. They are most often caused by improperly fitting shoes and socks; excessive hard use (such as in athletics); long standing or walking on hard surfaces; obesity or rapid weight gain (as in pregnancy); and improper weight-bearing through poor foot and leg alignment.

Exercises for the correction of postural deviations are generally based on the assumption that if it is a functional deformity, regardless of the factors causing the problem, muscular imbalance will be present.

If the muscles on one side of a joint are stronger than the muscles on the opposite side of that joint, then the body part is pulled in the direction of the stronger muscles. Corrective exercises are usually designed to strengthen the long, weak muscles and to stretch the short, strong ones in order to bring about an equal pull in both directions (see Concept 7).

Poor posture, especially lordosis, can cause back strain and pain and make the back more susceptible to injury. (196, 133)

The forward tilt of the pelvis may cause the sacral bone to press on nerve roots with consequent low back pain and sciatica. Some authorities advise the elimination of all exercises calling for the hyperextension of the spine for those with lordosis and weak abdominals. (91, 100, 101, 133) The incidence of lordosis is about the same among men and women. (93) There is added strain on the back during pregnancy. High heels contribute to spinal strain. (98, 105)

The neck is probably strained more frequently than the lower back.

The neck is constructed with the same curve and has the same mechanical problems as the lower back. The postural fault of "head forward" places a chronic strain on the posterior neck muscles that may cause referred pain to face, scalp, shoulder, arm and chest. (266, 277)

The overwhelming majority of back and neck aches are avoidable. A common cause of backache is muscular strain, frequently due to using the back improperly in daily activities or during exercise.

When lifting improperly there is great pressure on the lumbar discs and severe stress on the lumbar muscles and ligaments. Many popular exercises place great strain on the back (see Concept 18). Sleeping flat on the back or face on a soft mattress can cause lower back strain. (133, 277, 132, 98)

Muscular fatigue and weak muscles are frequent causes of backache.

Backache has been referred to as a "Hypokinetic Disease," meaning that it is caused by insufficient exercise. Lack of exercise results in weak muscles that are easily strained and fatigued. Sedentary workers are particularly susceptible to spinal strain, and weak abdominal and back muscles are especially to blame. If the abdominals are weak, the pelvis is apt to tilt forward, causing lordosis. (100, 166, 93, 105)

Most people agree excessive muscle tension is a contributing factor in painful spines.

Backaches may be triggered by worries, excitement, or fears; or by stimulation of already hypersensitive muscular areas, which have been referred to as "trigger points." These tender, painful spots occur frequently in the neck, shoulders, back, and hip as the result of constant tension, strain, or muscle spasm. When these tense muscles shorten, lose elasticity, and are weakened by lack of exercise, the "low back syndrome" occurs (see figure below).

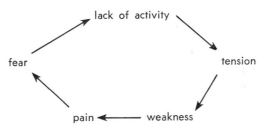

With a weak back, the mildest movement can trigger back pain. (228, 279) Back pains may result from "referred pain" from muscle tension in other areas. In some cases the pain is "referred" from the back of the legs if the hamstring muscles have been overstretched or injured.

There is no such thing as a "slipped disc."

Laymen frequently misunderstand disc problems. Vertebral discs may herniate or rupture, but they do not slip. Pressure of disc material on nerves causes pain and a protective reflex (muscle spasm) occurs to protect it. This causes more pain, thus a vicious cycle begins. The discs in the lumbar area are subjected to greater pressures, partly because they are at the bottom of the spine; therefore, they are more apt to be damaged by severe jolts or strains. (228, 93)

Most backaches can be prevented or alleviated by good sense and proper exercise.

Several "good sense" suggestions for taking care of the back are listed here. (75, 133, 228, 235, 134, 277, 98, 105)

1. Avoid the swayback position at all times by taking such precautions as the following:
    a. To relieve back strain during prolonged standing, try to keep the lower back flat by propping one foot on a stool, bar, or rail; alternate feet occasionally.
    b. When sitting, use a hard chair with a straight back and put the spine against it; keep one or both knees higher than the hips by crossing the legs (alternate sides) or using a foot rest, keeping the knees bent.
    c. When driving a car, place a hard seat-and-backrest combination over the seat of the automobile; pull the seat forward so the legs are bent when operating the pedals.
    d. When lying, keep the knees and hips bent; avoid lying on the abdomen; when lying on the back, a pillow or lift should be placed under the knees.
    e. Avoid lifting and carrying improperly (see Concept 13).
2. To prevent neck strain, avoid the head forward position. The forward thrust is apt to occur in such activities as card playing, sewing, studying, and watching television; sleeping on a high pillow may also cause back strain.
3. Do corrective exercises to strengthen the abdominal muscles and stretch the lower back muscles; avoid exercises that strain the lower back or cause it to arch.
4. General exercises, involving the entire body, are important in preventing weak muscles and lack of flexibility.
5. Warm up before engaging in strenuous activity.
6. Get adequate rest and sleep; avoid pushing yourself mentally or physically to the point of exhaustion.
7. Vary the working position by changing from one task to another before feeling fatigued; when doing desk work, get up and stretch occasionally to relieve tension.
8. Sleep on a firm mattress or place a three-fourths inch thick plywood board under the mattress.

9. Avoid sudden, jerky movements of the back.
10. The smaller the waistline, the lesser the strain on the lower back. Avoid being overweight.

Suggested Readings

Kelly, E. D. *Adapted and Corrective Physical Education,* 4th ed. New York: Ronald Press Co., 1965.

Michele, A. A. *Orthotherapy.* New York: M. Evans Company, Inc., 1971.

Mental and physical health are affected by an individual's ability to avoid or adapt to stress, emotional factors, and tension.

Stress, Tension, and Relaxation

14

Concept 14

Mental and physical health are affected by an individual's ability to avoid or adapt to stress, emotional factors, and tension.

Introduction

Stress can trigger an emotional response that in turn evokes the autonomic nervous system to a "fight or flight" response. This adaptive and protective device stimulates the ductless glands to hypo- or hyperactivity in preparation for what is perceived as a threat or assault on the whole organism. In some instances this "alarm reaction" of the body may be essential to survival, but when evoked inappropriately or excessively the adaptive reaction may be more harmful than the effects of the original stressor. (112, 279)

Terms

Adaptation—The body's efforts to restore normalcy.

Alarm Reaction—The body's warning signal that a stressor is present.

Anxiety—A state of apprehension with a compulsion to do something; excessive anxiety is a tension disorder with physiological characteristics. (81)

Chronic Fatigue—Constant state of fatigue in the entire body.

Neuromuscular Hypertension—Unnecessary or exaggerated muscle contractions; excess tension beyond that needed to perform a given task; also called hypertonus.

Physiological Fatigue—A deterioration in the capacity of the neuromuscular system as the result of physical overwork and strain; also referred to as "true fatigue."

Psychological Fatigue—A feeling of fatigue usually caused by such things as lack of exercise, boredom, or mental stress resulting in lack of energy and depression; also referred to as "subjective" or "false" fatigue.

Relaxation—The release or reduction of tension in the neuromuscular system.

Stress—The nonspecific response of the body to any demand made upon it. (247)

Stressor—Anything that produces stress or increases the rate of wear and tear on the body.

The Facts

All living creatures are in a continual state of stress (some more; some less). (279)

Stressors can be physical in nature or psychosocial. Physical stressors include heat, noise, overcrowding, malnutrition, climate, microorganisms, terrain, etc. (112, 279) Psychosocial stimuli are probably the most common stressors affecting humans. (247) These include "life-change events," such as change in work hours or line of work, family illnesses, problems with superiors, deaths of relatives or friends, and increased responsibilities. (112)

Too little stress is undesirable.

Stress is not always harmful. Moderate stress may enhance behavioral adaptation and is necessary for maturity and health. It stimulates psychological growth. (243) It has been said that "freedom from stress is death" and "stress is the spice of life." (247)

Too much stress or inability to adapt appropriately to stress is harmful.

Cumulative clinical evidence has demonstrated the linkage between stress and disease and death. (112) Mental and physical conditions that can result from psychosomatic causes (81) include high blood pressure and heart disease (14, 112), psychiatric disorders such as depression and schizophrenia (112), indigestion, colitis, ulcers, headaches, insomnia (137), diarrhea, constipation, increased blood clotting time, increased cholesterol concentration, diuresis, edema, low back pain, and others. (279)

Individuals react and adapt differently to different stressors.

What one person finds stressful may not be for others, and stress affects people differently. It mobilizes some to greater efficiency, while it confuses and disorganizes others.

An individual's response to stress depends upon the intensity of the threat, the type of situation in which it occurs and personal variables such as cultural background, tolerance levels, and past experience. (108, 112, 243, 279) The capacity of the individual to adapt is not a static function but fluctuates with his energy, drive, and courage. (279)

Individuals tend to adapt best to moderate stress.

One would expect mild stress to produce mild adaptations and strong stress to produce strong adaptive responses, but this is not so (see figure below). High levels of threat tend to evoke ineffective, disorganized behavior. (243)

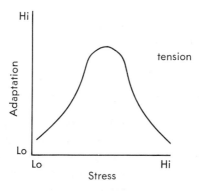

Stress can be self-induced and pleasurable or unpleasurable.

Some people may deliberately place themselves in stressful situations; for example, athletes place themselves under maximum strain; lawyers and surgeons are challenged by difficulties; pregnancy imposes psychological and physiological stress on a woman. Self-induced stress may also be an unpleasant but necessary interlude that cannot be avoided. For example, there is a risk of falling that is necessary to learn to ride a bicycle. (243)

Neuromuscular hypertension may be both a cause and an effect of stress.

Tension is a primary index of stress (see figure). (243) Anxiety is an emotional response caused by stressors that can be seen in the form of muscular tension. (81) Muscular tension may also be physical in origin, resulting from overuse of a muscle group. This tension can cause muscle spasms and pain that in turn become additional stressors. (243, 279, 280)

Excessive tension can cause psychophysical disorders.

One physician claims 50 percent of his patients have tension disorders. They are of three types: (a) primary—those caused by tension (irritable colon, spastic esophogus, nervousness, emotional imbalance, fatigue, insomnia, etc.); (b) mixed—those that probably would not have occurred in the absence of hypertonus (high blood pressure, peptic ulcers, angina, etc.); and (c) secondary—those in which tension is the result of pain and discomfort from other conditions such as fractures and tumors. (138)

Some tension is normally present in muscles and contributes to the adjustment of the individual to his environment.

We need some tension to remain awake, alert, and ready to respond—a certain degree aids some types of mental activity. There appears to be an optimum level of tension for each individual to facilitate the thought process. However, too much tension can inhibit some types of mental activity and physical skills (such as those requiring accuracy and steadiness in held postures). (181, 224)

Fatigue and neuromuscular hypertension are closely related.

High levels of tension are a source of fatigue. Fatigue from lack of rest, sleep, emotional strain, pain, disease, and muscular work may produce too much muscle tension. Fatigue may be either psychological or physiological in origin, but both can result in a state of exhaustion or chronic fatigue with muscle tenseness. (137, 138, 224)

Excessive tension can be avoided or relieved by proper planning of our daily lives.

"Moderation in all things" may still be a helpful adage. Work must be balanced with rest. Provision should be made for recreational activities and diversions. Diversions may be even more important than rest, since stress on one system helps to relax another. This may range from a temporary change from one task to another (e.g., from studying to lawn mowing) or a change of scene, a change in job, a vacation, or even retirement. (154, 224, 247, 279) We may even need to change our approach to life.

Some methods of relieving tension are less desirable or not recommended.

There is no magic cure for stress or tension, but there are a variety of therapeutic approaches. Hypnosis may lead to fantasy and dependency. Alcoholic beverages, tranquilizers, and painkillers may give temporary relief and may be prescribed by the physician as a part of the treatment, but they do not relieve the cause of the problem and may even mask the symptoms or cause further problems. Chemotherapy does not provide a long-term solution to chronic tension; neither does another treatment: the drastic surgery called a frontal lobotomy!

Mild rhythmic exercises, stretching exercises, heat, and massage are beneficial in relaxing "tight" muscles. In some cases, group therapy and counseling have been used successfully in alleviating the causes of anxiety and tension. (138, 154, 224)

There are several satisfactory methods of releasing tension through techniques of conscious relaxation.

In some way not fully understood, certain involuntary bodily functions can be controlled by an act of will (voluntarily). Relaxation of the muscles is a skill that can be learned through practice just as other muscle skills are learned. (14, 137, 138)

Conscious relaxation techniques usually employ the "Three R's" of relaxation: (1) Reduce mental activity, (2) Recognize tension, and (3) Reduce respiration.

Some examples of these systems are described below:

A. *Jacobson's Progressive Relaxation Method*—One must recognize how a tense muscle feels before one can voluntarily release the tension. In this technique, the individual contracts the muscles strongly and then relaxes. Each of the large muscles is relaxed and later the small ones. The contractions are gradually reduced in intensity until no movement is visible. Always, the emphasis is placed on detecting the feeling of tension as the first step in "letting go," or "going negative." Jacobson emphasizes the importance of relaxing eye muscles and speech muscles, since he believes these muscles trigger reactions of the total organism more than other muscles. (148, 149)

B. *Autogenic (self-generated) Relaxation Training*—Relaxation is brought about by passive concentration upon phrases of preselected words. This practice is done several times daily, lying down in a quiet room with eyes closed. This technique has been used to focus on heaviness of limbs, warmth of limbs, heart regulation, breathing regulation, and coolness in the forehead. It evokes changes opposite to those produced by stress. (11, 239, 244)

C. *Biofeedback-Autogenic Relaxation Training*—Biofeedback training utilizes machines that monitor certain physiological processes of the body and provide visual or auditory evidence of what is happening to normally unconscious bodily functions. When combined with autogenic phrases, subjects have learned to relax and reduce the electrical activity in their muscles, lower blood pressure by increasing the temperature of their hands, and decrease headaches, asthma attacks, and other psychosomatic disorders. (11, 104, 230, 239)

D. *Yoga and TM*—Transcendental meditation has been practiced for years in India, but need not be associated with a formal religion. Like autogenic training, these techniques are done in a quiet atmosphere. The individual assumes a comfortable sitting position and attempts to block out distracting thoughts by mentally repeating a personal secret word or phrase. In addition to meditation, many of the yoga stretching exercises are helpful in relaxing tension of specific muscle groups. Research has shown that those skilled in this technique can decrease their oxygen consumption, change the electrical activity of the brain, slow the metabolism, decrease blood lactate, lower body temperature, and slow the heart rate. (14, 40)

E. *Imagery*—Along with autogenic phrases, one can visualize such feelings as "sinking into a mattress or pillow" or can think of being a "limp, loose-jointed puppet with no one to hold the strings." One can imagine being a "half-filled sack of flour resting on an uneven surface" or pretend to be "a sack of granulated salt left out in the rain and melting away." Some people seem to respond better to the concept of "floating" rather than of feeling "heavy," but whatever the image that one wishes to conjure, it is a form of self-hypnosis that helps to take the mind off anxieties and distractions and at the same time allows the release of unwanted tensions in the muscles through "mind over matter." (154)

F. *Tension Relieving Exercises*—Some specific but simple tension relieving exercises that can be used with little previous "muscle relaxing" experience are presented in Lab 24.

Suggested Readings

Benson, H. *The Relaxation Response.* New York: William Morrow and Company, Inc., 1975.

Fried, J. "Biofeedback: Teaching Your Body to Heal Itself," *Family Health,* Feb. 1974; and *Reader's Digest,* May 1974, p. 110.

Jacobson, E. *Anxiety and Tension Control.* Philadelphia: J. B. Lippincott Company, 1964.

Wolff, H. G. *Stress and Disease,* 2d ed. Edited by S. Wolf and H. Goodell. Springfield, Ill.: Charles C Thomas, Publisher, 1968.

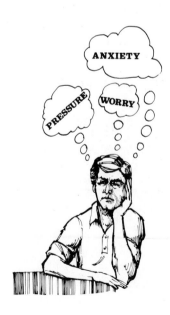

The contribution of regular exercise to physical and mental fitness makes it an important factor in good health.

Health and Physical Activity

15

Concept 15

The contribution of regular exercise to physical and mental fitness makes it an important factor in good health.

Introduction

Man responds to the environment as a whole—as a total human being. There is no such thing as independent physical health and mental health. A person's physical well-being affects mental health and vice versa. So interrelated and integrated are the parts that anything that affects one part brings about changes in others. Thus, since one's health is composed of many components, the proper development and function of each component is necessary for an overall sound level of health.

The Facts

Health is more than freedom from disease.

Since health is a complex, ever-changing phenomenon, it is not surprising that the concept of health has undergone change. Previously, health was considered the crown on the well man's head that only the sick man could see. This interpretation of health has evolved to the following definitions of health:

1. "Health is a state of complete physical, mental, and social well-being and not merely the absence of disease and infirmity." (197)
2. "Health is personal fitness for full, fruitful, enjoyable living." (130)
3. "Health is more than the absence of disease, defect, disability, pain or decay; it encompasses the presence of vigor and vitality, social well-being, and a zest for living." (130)

Optimal health includes sound mental health, good physical fitness, and an established spiritual faith or personal philosophy. (130)

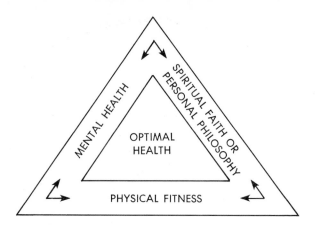

Personal health has been depicted as a triangle with three interrelated dimensions: physical fitness, mental health, and spiritual faith or personal philosophy. (130) These components combine to form optimal health. The concept of health has shifted from the negative view (lack of certain aspects) to a positive outlook (possession of certain attributes).

Regular physical activity can contribute to the achievement of physical fitness, which is one of the important components of good health.

Many of the important benefits of regular physical activity to good health and physical fitness have already been described elsewhere in this book. A summary of some of the major benefits of regular physical activity is presented in Table 15.1.

Participation in regular physical activity can contribute to mental health, which is one of the important components of good health.

Just as the concept of health has changed, so has the concept of mental health. Mental illness is now recognized as a health problem and not a personal weakness or reason for social disgrace. The serious nature of mental health problems is illustrated by the following facts: approximately twenty-five thousand suicides occur in this country each year; (252); doctors estimate that as many as 70 percent of all illnesses are psychosomatic or emotionally related (197); statistics show dramatic increases in cost for care of those with mental illnesses. (5)

Physical activity contributes to physical fitness and sound physical health but also contributes to sound mental health. Some of the benefits to mental health derived from regular physical activity are summarized in Table 15.2.

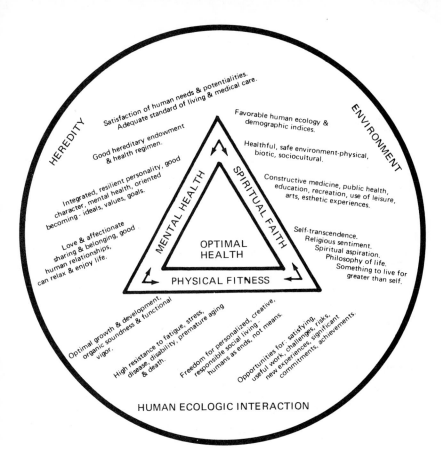

Factors and conditions related to our modern theoretical concepts of optimal health.

Regular exercise is very beneficial, but it is not a panacea.

While research does support many values of exercise, it is not a cure-all. For example, there is no evidence that exercise can reduce viral or bacterial infection. Accordingly, each person should carefully evaluate all claims before making exercise decisions.

The choices one makes (behavior) during a lifetime are the most decisive factors in reaching optimal health.

We are repeatedly faced with the need to make decisions about our health. Our good health depends on the decisions we make. Just as we must decide what foods to eat, whether to listen to the doctor or not, or whether to smoke or not; we must also make the decision as to whether or not we will exercise regularly. The decisions of when and how to exercise will determine the benefits that will be realized in the form of good or optimal health.

Table 15.1 The Physical Health Benefits of Activity

Major Benefit	Related Benefits
Improved Cardiovascular Fitness	• stronger heart muscle • lower heart rate • possible reduction in blood pressure • reduced blood fat • possible resistance to atherosclerosis • possible improved peripheral circulation • improved coronary circulation • resistance to "emotional storm" • less chance of heart attack • greater chance of surviving a heart attack
Greater Lean Body Mass and Lesser Body Fat	• greater work efficiency • less succeptibility to disease • improved appearance • less incidence of self-concept problems related to obesity
Improved Strength and Muscular Endurance	• greater work efficiency • less chance of muscle injury • decreased chance of low back problems • improved performance in sports • improved ability to meet emergencies
Improved Flexibility	• greater work efficiency • less chance of muscle injury • less chance of joint injury • decreased chance of low back problems • improved sports performance
Other Health Benefits of Exercise and Physical Activity	• increased ability to use oxygen • quicker recovery after hard work • delay in the aging process • greater respiratory efficiency • possible increase in efficiency of the vital organs other than the heart and muscles. • decreased muscle tension

Table 15.2 The Mental Health Benefits of Activity

Major Benefit	Related Benefits
Reduction in Mental Tension	• fewer stress symptoms • ability to enjoy leisure • possible work improvement
Opportunity for Social Interactions	• improved quality of life
Resistence to Fatigue	• ability to enjoy leisure • improved quality of life • improved ability to meet some stressors
Opportunity for Successful Experience	• improved self-concept • opportunity to recognize and accept personal limitations
Improved Physical Fitness	• improved sense of well-being • improved self-concept • improved appearance

Suggested Readings

deVries, H. A. *Physiology of Exercise: For Physical Education and Athletics.* Dubuque, Iowa: Wm. C. Brown Company Publishers, 1974.

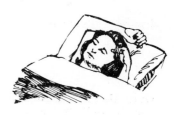

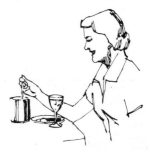

Physical education is more than just physical fitness and health.

Psychosocial Considerations

Concept 16

Physical education is more than just physical fitness and health.

Introduction

Much has been said in recent years about the psychosocial "values" of physical activity and sport. In fact, many claims have been made that are difficult to verify. It is not the purpose of this unit to review these "marginal" claims but to present some facts that might be helpful to persons interested in continuing physical activity throughout life. While basic social and psychological patterns are almost entirely established by the college or adult years, there are some psychosocial considerations concerning physical activity that should be meaningful to adults. This unit is designed to present some of these facts.

Terms

Aesthetic—The theory, study, or appreciation of beautiful things.

Catharsis—The release or purifying of one's emotions; for the purposes of this book, the release of stress and tension.

Movement Personality—An individual's characteristic way of moving.

Psychosocial—In this book the term is used to characterize factors related to the individual's behavior (alone or as a member of a group) specifically with reference to sport and physical activity.

The Facts

Movement has meaning. (195)

As discussed in previous chapters, movement is a means to many ends. Through movement one performs work, achieves health and physical fitness, and accomplishes other useful objectives. However, movement can be an end in itself. Those who have performed a dance, played a game, or jogged a mile realize that the mere performance of these tasks are accomplishments in themselves. Movement and physical activity does not always have to be purposeful; satisfaction can be derived from the mere involvement in a movement experience.

There are at least seven major reasons why people participate in regular physical activity. (156, 157, 88)

People participate in activity for different reasons. Some of these reasons are listed below.

1. Physical activity for social purpose. People may choose activity for their own social enjoyment or as a means of advancing socially.
2. Physical activity for thrills and excitement. People seek excitement and certain types of activities can fulfill man's need for excitement.
3. Physical activity for aesthetic experience. Some forms of activity are more aesthetic or beautiful than others. Participation in dance or an individual sport such as gymnastics can be a beautiful experience both for the participant and the observer.
4. Physical activity for recreation and relaxation. In an age of stress and tension some people choose to be active as a means of relaxing and relieving tensions. Various activities can provide a means of getting away from it all, blowing off steam, or venting frustrations in a socially acceptable manner.
5. Physical activity to meet a challenge. Some people enjoy the challenge of vigorous training and physical accomplishments. Marathon runners reap satisfaction from completing the race, football players enjoy contact, and race drivers relish the danger of racing. Meeting a challenge is one reason why people engage in regular physical activity.
6. Physical activity as games of chance. There are some who participate in activity, though not commonly of a vigorous nature, to determine their ability to pick a winner. For these people, chance or the luck involved in the activity is the major reason for their participation. Dice and horse racing are examples of this type of activity. (157)
7. Physical activity as a means of achieving health and physical fitness. The most common reason why people participate in physical activity is to improve their physical fitness and health.

People choose recreational activities in which they succeed. (41)

Most men and women will choose leisure activities in which they enjoy success. Every individual should develop skills in "lifetime" sports to insure success in recreational pursuits later in life.

Success in lifetime sports need not be equated with "winning." (99)

Sport psychologists agree that one problem experienced by many Americans in sport is that they cannot enjoy sports unless they "win." The chances of success and enjoyment of sports, especially of the competitive variety increases with the realization that success is not necessarily equated with winning. Though most people who play sports enjoy winning, it must be realized that only 50 percent of the participants can win a given contest. Suggestions for finding success and enjoyment in sport are listed below:

1. Set realistic goals for yourself. To play well against someone better than you should be considered a successful experience.
2. Consider a handicap system such as that used in golf or bowling.
3. In team sports or doubles games, change partners frequently to make competition more balanced.
4. Consider, before you play, the benefits you expect to get from participation—social contact, release of tension, physical fitness—if these are accomplished you have been successful.
5. Consider your improvement over a period of time as your successful accomplishment.
6. Consider the fun of playing as your success and don't allow a "poor score" (compared to an opponent's) to take the fun away.
7. If you cannot have fun unless you win the game, consider noncompetitive activities such as jogging, swimming, bicycling, etc.

Overemphasis in sport and physical activity can detract from enjoyment of the activity and can create anxiety in the performer.

Whatever the benefits of regular physical activity or sport, none should be exaggerated to the point of detracting from a fuller life. There is evidence that overemphasis on sports can cause anxiety and even a type of neurosis. (183)

To be a spectator at a sports event is NOT NECESSARILY bad.

There is little doubt that there is a danger in our society of watching rather than doing. This is especially dangerous if an individual is *always* a spectator and never a participant. However, to enjoy watching sports could be compared to enjoying a form of art. Steinhaus (259) likens the performance of a sports team to "creating a picture of the highest form of art." He believes that sport and art can bring to man "a satisfying experience" and be a "transmitter of culture."

Involvement in regular physical activity can benefit a person socially and emotionally.

Although some recent studies have indicated that participation in highly competitive athletics may not contribute to character development (209) or good sportsmanship (64), there is evidence that those people involved in regular exercise throughout life reap both social and emotional benefits.

1. Participation in physical activity can provide a "catharsis" or emotional release from the pent-up tensions of regular daily activity. (178)
2. Physically fit individuals are more likely to try new leisure activities that can provide for a meaningful social life. (68)
3. People who exercise regularly are more likely to have good physical health, which is a contributor to good total health including good mental health. (68)

Whatever psychosocial benefits sport and physical activity have for men, they also have for women.

In the past, sport was the domain of men, with women relegated to a role of spectator. Much of the reason for this was related to the ideas that women were "too emotional" to participate in competitive activities or that it was unfeminine. There is no research to indicate that sports programs with good leadership are harmful to women. In fact, women can and do benefit from regular physical activity in the same ways as male participants, and it is now a culturally acceptable and popular program for women. (170)

Just as each person has an individual personality, one also has a unique movement personality. (95, 131)

No two people move in the same way. (131) Given similar circumstances, different people react with different movement patterns according to their personalities. One's movement can convey his personality and communicate his feelings! Because movement personalities differ there is wide variety in the leisure activities selected by different individuals. People should try to select leisure activities that are compatible with their own movement personalities.

Suggested Readings

Ellis, M. J. *Why People Play*. Englewood Cliffs, N. J.: Prentice-Hall, 1973.
Leonard, G. *The Ultimate Athlete*. New York: The Viking Press, 1974.
Landers, D. M., ed. *Social Problems in Athletics*. Urbana, Ill.: The University of Illinois Press, 1976.
Scott, J. *The Athletic Revolution*. New York: The Free Press, 1971.
Gerber, E. W., et al. *The American Woman in Sport*. Reading, Mass.: Addison-Wesley, 1974.

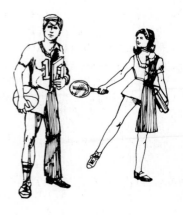

There are many different exercises, both formal and informal, that can be adapted to the needs of individuals.

Programs of Exercise 17

Concept 17

There are many different exercises, both formal and informal, that can be adapted to the needs of individuals.

Introduction

Over the years many different types of exercise programs have been developed with the intent of meeting the needs of people of diverse interests and needs. Among the more popular and well-known exercise programs are: The Aerobics Program, the President's Council on Physical Fitness and Sports Adult Fitness Program, the Royal Canadian XBX and 5BX Programs, Continuous Rhythmical Exercise, Circuit Training, Interval Training, Jogging, Aerobic Dance, Weight Training, Calisthenics, and Sports Exercise Programs. Each of these programs is described briefly and a brief analysis of the strengths and weakness of each is presented so that the reader can consider the possibility of using one of these plans as part of a personal physical activity program.

Terms

Formal Exercise Program—A program that is preplanned and done to predetermined specifications.

Informal Exercise Program—Informal exercise is done without a formalized plan and is frequently done "on one's own" as opposed to being part of a class or group.

Programs of Exercise

Aerobics: Based on the needs of military personnel, Dr. Kenneth Cooper developed a program of physical fitness that he called Aerobics. Aerobics means "with oxygen." Basically, exercises are of two types: aerobic, those that can be performed with the amount of oxygen the body can supply; and anaerobic, those that are so vigorous that the body does not supply the muscles with enough oxygen to continue work. In anaerobic exercise the body incurs an oxygen "debt" as exercise continues. The "debt" is paid back after exercise. For example, the 100-yard dash is anaerobic. During the run the body requires more oxygen than is supplied. After the run the heart rate and rate of breathing remain high to pay back the "debt." Cooper suggests that physical fitness is best developed in aerobic activities or those activities that can be continued for a long time without building up an oxygen debt.

In the Aerobics program several activities are suggested as methods for developing physical fitness. Each activity is selected according to the amount of oxygen required to perform the activity. The more oxygen a person uses to perform the activity, the greater the likelihood that the activity will actually contribute to physical fitness. Each of the activities is assigned a point value on the basis of its oxygen consumption and its ability to produce physical fitness.

In order to reap the cardiovascular benefits of the Aerobics program, an individual must earn thirty points a week by performing any combination of the activities suggested. Details of the program are outlined in Appendix 3, page 270.

Although the program of Aerobics was developed for use by air force personnel, it has received wide recognition as a method of physical fitness development for the average American. (For complete details on the program refer to the Suggested Readings.)

Adult Physical Fitness Program: The President's Council on Physical Fitness and Sports, because of its concern for the total physical fitness of every American, has developed a program of progressive exercise that can be adapted to the specific needs of the individual. A sample program is presented in Appendix 4, page 272. (For more details refer to the Suggested Readings.)

Royal Canadian XBX and 5BX Programs: The XBX program and the 5BX program are programs of progressive exercise designed to build total physical fitness. These plans, originally developed for use by The Royal Canadian Air Force, require eleven to twelve minutes a day. They were, like the Aerobics program, originally designed as programs for developing and maintaining the physical fitness of military personnel. However, the programs have been widely received by the public. The exercises are progressive in nature and the intensity of exercise is graduated according to the fitness level of the individual performing them. A sample program is presented in Appendix 5, page 274. (For more details refer to the Suggested Readings.)

Continuous Rhythmical Exercise: This type of exercise program was pioneered by Dr. Thomas Cureton at the University of Illinois. Each person progresses at his or her own rate or ability from low intensity exercise to exercise of higher intensity. Cureton labeled the different stages low gear, middle gear, and high gear. Every lesson begins with an introduction, a warm-up period, the main exercises, and a tapering off period involving deep breathing, stretching, massage, and rest. Work is continuous with a build-up of speed and exertion during each lesson. The low-gear program emphasizes flexibility and endurance exercises conducted at a slow pace. The middle-gear exercises are more difficult exercises performed at a faster pace and for a longer period of time. Emphasis is on flexibility, strength, and endurance. The high-gear program consists of high speed exercises designed to place greater demands on the body in terms of strength, endurance, flexibility, balance, speed, and power. A modified continuous rhythmical endurance program is presented in Appendix 6, page 278. (The reader is referred to the suggested readings by Cureton and Corbin for further details.)

Circuit Training: This is a physical training program of timed exercises at several stations. Each day a participant is to complete the series of exercise stations (placed around a gymnasium or field) in a shorter time. Each station may require several repetitions of an activity such as pull-ups, squat thrusts, push-ups, medicine ball put, agility run, and sit-ups. The circuit may consist of an obstacle course of various activities including climbing, crawling, running, and lifting. After correctly completing each exercise the performer moves on to the next station attempting to complete the circuit as quickly as possible. The objective is to complete the circuit in less time on each successive day. At intervals the number of repetitions or the difficulty of the activities is increased. A sample Circuit Training Program is presented in Appendix 7, page 280. (For more information the reader is referred to the reading by Morgan and Adamson in the Suggested Readings.)

Speed Play or Fartlek: Fartlek is a Swedish word for Speed Play. This type of exercise was developed in Scandinavia where pinewood paths follow curves of lakes, up and down many hills where the scenery takes one's mind off the task at hand. The idea is to get away from the regimen of running on a track and enjoy the woods, lakes, and mountains. Because of the terrain the pace is never constant, since the uphill path requires a slowing down while a straight stretch or downhill trail allows for speed. In the speed play or system one runs easily for a time, a steady hard speed for a while, rapid walking, easy running broken with wind-sprints, full speed uphill, and a fast pace for a while. A sample program is presented in Appendix 8, page 282. (For more information refer to the suggested reading by Wilt.)

Interval Training Program: An interval training program is a running program of repeated anaerobic running or swimming for short periods of time separated by measured intervals of recovery jogging or stroking. (As developed by Gerschler of Germany, the stress of anaerobic running raises the heart rate to near maximal from which it drops to 110-120 during recovery.) This program is controlled in terms of distance, pace, number of repetitions, and recovery interval, allowing for a wide variety of programs at various intensities. Guidelines for this type of intermittent training are presented in the discussion of anaerobic training on page 17. (The reader is referred to the suggested readings by Wilt and Astrand for further details.) A sample program is presented in Appendix 9, p. 283.

Jogging Program: It is generally recommended that a jogging program begin slowly, alternating walking and jogging a quarter-mile, and gradually building up to a mile or more at such a speed that you can talk easily to another person as you run. Intensity, frequency, and duration of jogging can be varied according to needs of specific individuals. The heart rate can be used to determine the desired intensity of exercise for a jogging program. The reader is referred to the aerobic exercise guidelines on page 17 for details. A sample jogging plan is presented in Appendix 10, page 284. (Additional information on jogging can be found in the Suggested Readings by Sheehan and Clarke.)

Aerobic Dance: Aerobic Dance is a modification of aerobics that includes some calisthenics and some basic dance or rhythmical steps. Developed by Jackie Sorenson, Aerobic Dance was designed to increase cardiovascular fitness through sustained aerobic exercise, but it was also designed to create interest for those people who enjoyed dancing and moving to music as opposed to running or jogging. In Aerobic Dance the participant alternately performs dance steps, jogging in place, and calisthenics. (For further details the reader is referred to the suggested reading by Sorenson.)

Weight Training: Weight training is performed using barbells, dumbells, pulleys, or other types of weight machines. Generally, weight training is performed isotonically. However, it can be modified to include isometric contractions. Weight "lifting" is *not* the same thing as weight "training." Weight training is exercising to improve your fitness level while weight lifting is an international sport that involves competition in three basic lifts. Information relating to weight training (isotonic and isometric exercise) is presented on pages 34 and 35. In addition the reader is referred to Appendix 11, page 285 and Appendix 12, page 289.

Calisthenics: Calisthenics are programs consisting of a series of formal exercises. Actually, the Adult Fitness Programs, the XBX, and the 5BX programs are calisthenic programs. A calisthenic program can be adapted to individual needs by selecting the exercises of your choice. The reader could develop a program of calisthenics by selecting exercises from Labs 22, 26, 27, 28, 35 and 36.

Sports Exercise Programs: Because sports and games are often fun and enjoyable many people choose them as their form of regular exercise. While some sports require considerable activity and are quite good for developing physical fitness, not all sports and games are active enough to promote physical fitness. Activities such as bowling, softball, and even golf are often not vigorous enough to build or maintain reasonable levels of physical fitness in young adults. Sports do have many advantages, but one should consider supplementing a sports exercise program with some other more vigorous type of activity if physical fitness is the goal. An advantage of sports and games as a regular form of exercise is the wide variety of activities from which the participant can select. Information concerning the value of different sports for physical fitness development is presented in Lab. 37, page 249.

There are advantages and disadvantages of each of the various types of exercise programs.

Since the needs and interests of each individual are unique, it is obvious that no single exercise program is best suited for all individuals. One should study each of the different programs and select the program (or combination of programs) that is best for that individual. Some of the advantages and disadvantages of each of the programs are presented in Table 17.1 on the following page. IT SHOULD BE EMPHASIZED THAT THE ADVANTAGES OR DISADVANTAGES OF ANY SPECIFIC PROGRAM DEPEND ON THE NEEDS AND INTERESTS OF A GIVEN INDIVIDUAL. FOR THIS REASON THE INFORMATION PRESENTED IN TABLE 17.1 MAY NOT BE ENTIRELY ACCURATE FOR ALL INDIVIDUALS. THE TABLE ATTEMPTS TO SUMMARIZE THE INFORMATION BASED ON THE NEEDS AND INTERESTS OF THE "TYPICAL AMERICAN."

Suggested Readings

Astrand, P. O. and K. Rodahl. *Textbook of Work Physiology*. New York: McGraw-Hill, 1970.

Clarke, H. H., ed. "Jogging." *Physical Fitness Research Digest*. 7(1):1-23, 1977.

Cooper, K. H. *The New Aerobics*. New York: M. Evans Co., 1970.

——"Key to Fitness at Any Age—The New Aerobics," *The Reader's Digest*. March 1970, pp. 213-230.

—— and Cooper, M. *Aerobics for Women*. New York: M. Evans Co., 1972.

Key
++ Good
+ Fair
— Poor

Table 17.1 Strengths and Weaknesses of Various Exercise Programs

Program Type	Cardiovascular fitness	Strength and muscular endurance	Flexibility	Body and fat control	Skill related fitness	Enjoyment or fun*
Aerobics	++	—	—	++	—	+
Adult Fitness Program	—	++	++	+	—	—
XBX-5BX	—	++	++	+	—	—
Rhythmical Endurance	++	++	++	++	—	+
Circuit Training	++	++	++	++	—	+
Speed Play or Fartlek	++	+	—	++	—	+
Interval Training	++	+	—	++	—	+
Jogging	++	+	—	++	—	+
Aerobic Dance	++	+	++	++	+	++
Weight Training	—	++	+	+	—	+
Calisthenics	—	++	++	+	—	—
Sports	**	**	**	**	++	++

*Enjoyment and fun are relative and for this reason it is impossible to classify activities accurately. However, for the average person some activities seem to be more enjoyable than others. The above listed classifications reflect the opinions of the typical person. ANY OF THE ACTIVITIES LISTED ABOVE CAN BE FUN AND ENJOYABLE FOR A GIVEN PERSON IN THE RIGHT CIRCUMSTANCES.

**Since the nature of different sports determines the value of that sport it must be said that this benefit may or may not be developed in sport.

Corbin, C. B. "An Exercise Program for Large Groups," *The Physical Educator*. 30:46, March 1973.

Cureton, T. K. *Physical Fitness and Dynamic Health*. New York: Dial Press, 1965.

Fox, E. L. and Mathews, D. K. *Interval Training*. Philadelphia: Saunders, 1974.

Morgan, R. and G. T. Adamson. *Circuit Training*. New Rochelle, N. Y.: Sportshelf and Soccer Associates, 1961.

President's Council on Physical Fitness. *Adult Physical Fitness*. Washington, D. C.: U.S. Government Printing Office, publication No. 20402. Copies available from Superintendent of Documents.

Royal Canadian Air Force. *Exercise Plans for Physical Fitness*. Queen's Printer, Ottawa, Canada; Revised U.S. Edition, published by Simon and Schuster, Inc., by special arrangement with *This Week Magazine*. Copies available from *This Week Magazine*, P. O. Box 77-E, Mount Vernon, N. Y.

Sheehan, George A. *Dr. Sheehan on Running*. Mountain View, Calif.: World Publications, 1975.

Sorensen, J. *Have Fun! Keep Fit!* LP1120 Booklet, available from Educational Activities Inc., Box 392, Freeport, N. Y.

Wilt, F. "Training for Competitive Running." In *Exercise Physiology*. Falls, H. B., ed. New York: Academic Press, 1968, chap. 14.

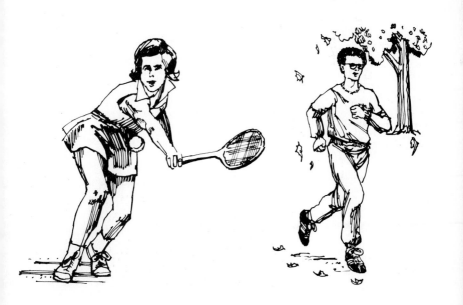

There are correct and incorrect ways to exercise. For maximum benefits, one should know the difference between the facts and the fallacies.

Exercise Cautions and Fallacies

18

Concept 18

There are correct and incorrect ways to exercise. For maximum benefits, one should know the difference between the facts and the fallacies.

Introduction

Mankind has always searched for the "easy," the "quick," and the "miraculous" route to health and happiness. This search has included the areas of physical fitness, especially exercise and weight loss. Because of the popularity of these two subjects, the mass media have made it possible to convey as much *mis*information as information. Everyone should seek the truth. This chapter attempts to expose some myths and separate fact from fallacy.

Terms

Hyperventilation—"Over-breathing"; forced rapid or deep-breathing.
I.U.D.—Intrauterine device for birth control.
Lumbar—Lower back region.
Synnovial Membrane—The membrane surrounding the freely movable joints in the body.
Valsalva Maneuver—Exerting force with the glottis closed, increasing intrathoracic pressure and raising arterial pressure. When released, arterial pressure drops rapidly, blood vessels expand and then are filled, causing a lag in blood flow to the left ventricle; thus, peripheral arterial blood pressure drops.

The Facts

Exercise has many benefits, but it is not a panacea. (181)

There are many benefits of exercise described throughout this book, but for those who contemplate beginning a fitness or reducing program, these reminders are included: (A) the most satisfactory way to lose weight is a combination of caloric reduction and exercise; (B) exercise will not change the size of boney structures (e.g., ankles); (C) exercise will not change the size of glands (e.g., women's breasts are glands; bust *girth* may be increased by developing chest *muscles*); (D) exercise does not "break-up" fatty deposits, but it does burn calories and thus, eventually, fat; (E) exercise does not *insure* good posture or good health, but it does help to attain and maintain it; and (F) there is no such thing as effortless exercise.

Passive exercise is NOT effective in weight reduction, spot reduction, increasing strength, or increasing endurance. (180)

Passive exercises come in a variety of forms, some of which are described below:

1. Rolling Machines—These ineffective wooden or metal rollers, moved by an electric motor, roll up and down the body part to which they are applied.

2. Vibrating Belts—These wide canvas or leather belts may be designed for the chin or for the hips, thighs, and abdomen. Driven by an electric motor, they jerk back and forth causing loose tissue of the body part to shake. They do *not* "break down" fat nor are they effective in weight loss or reduction of girth. (123, 147) These devices may cause a temporary increase in local circulation, but they may also be potentially harmful if used on the abdomen, especially if used by women during pregnancy, menstruation, or while an I.U.D. is in place. (180)

3. Vibrating Tables and Pillows—Contrary to advertisements, these passive devices will *not* improve posture, trim the figure, reduce the weight, or develop muscle tonus. They may be useful in inducing relaxation.

4. Motor Driven Cycles and Rowing Machines—Like all mechanical devices that "do the work" for the individual, these machines are *not* effective in weight reduction, figure improvement, or development of physical fitness. They may help increase circulation and flexibility. Only if the rider exerts his own effort against the machine by opposing or hurrying its rhythm could some beneficial strengthening be expected to occur. (180)

5. Massage—Whether done by a masseur or by a mechanical device, massage is passive, requiring no effort on the part of the individual. It can help increase circulation, prevent or loosen adhesions, and induce relaxation, but it has *no* value in developing physical fitness or in removing fatty tissue. (180)

6. Electric Muscle Stimulators—These devices when applied to a muscle, cause the muscle to contract involuntarily. They are dangerous in that

they may induce heart attacks; complicate gastrointestinal, ortho-pedic, kidney, and other disorders; and possibly aggravate epilepsy, hernia, varicose veins, etc. In the hands of qualified medical personnel, muscle stimulators are valuable therapeutic devices. They should never be used by the layman and have no place in a reducing or fitness program. (251)

7. Weighted Belts—These belts are claimed to reduce waists, thighs, and hips when worn for several hours under one's clothing. In reality, they do none of these things and have been reported to cause actual phys-ical harm. (251)

8. Inflated Belts, Inflated Shorts, and Sauna Suits—The rubberized in-flated devices are sometimes referred to as "Sauna Belts or Shorts." The "suits" are air-tight plastic or rubberized garments. Evidence in-dicates that their claims of girth reducing are unwarranted. If one performs exercise in conjunction with the wearing of such garments, the exercise (*not* the garment) may have beneficial effects. (251)

9. Figure Wrapping—Some reducing salons advertise that wrapping the body in bandages soaked in a "magic solution" will cause a perma-nent reduction in body girth. This so-called "treatment" is pure quack-ery. There is no magic solution that will make fat disappear and the pressure of the bandages can at best have a very temporary shrink-ing effect (the way one's watch band may temporarily indent the arm). (182) It may be dangerous to your health.

Some active exercises should be used with caution or not used at all by some individuals, and some popular exercises do not have the benefits commonly ascribed to them.

A few such exercises are described here.

1. Double Leg Lifts—Raising and lowering both legs simultaneously from the back-lying position is a potentially dangerous exercise for the per-son with weak abdominals. This exercise is often mistakenly pre-scribed for strengthening the abdominals, but it is in reality a hip flexor exercise. If the abdominals are not well developed, the pull of the hip flexor muscles on the pelvis and lumbar spine will cause the back to arch during the exercise. This may result in serious injury to the back. In addition, it will further stretch the already weakened abdominals and possibly cause an abdominal hernia. (6, 171, 181, 185, 255)

2. Sit-up with Straight Legs—This exercise has the same effect as double leg-lifts in terms of the anatomical and mechanical stresses involved. It is primarily an exercise for the muscles that flex the hip joint. If

weak abdominals are present and the lower back is permitted to hyperextend, injury may result. Sit-ups are best performed with the knees bent and the feet unstabilized; the spine should "curl" up and "curl" down.

3. Deep Knee Bends—Deep squatting exercises may be harmful to the knee joint, causing a stretching of the ligaments and an irritation of the synovial membrane. (73, 159, 171, 185) If one desires to strengthen the legs by knee bends, the half-squat (with a 90° angle of knee flexion) is a satisfactory substitute.

4. Backbends—The acrobatic backbend and other exercises such as the "swan" position and backward trunk circling that require arching the lower back are designed to increase the strength of the lumbar muscles or increase trunk flexibility. For the individual who has weak abdominals and/or "sway back," such exercises further aggravate these conditions. (237)

5. Standing Toe Touches—Some people, because of body build may never be able to touch their toes, but they have strived mightily by vigorous "bounces" of up to 100 repetitions! The exercise is controversial, but because of the potential for abuse and the possibility of gravity-assisted momentum causing injury to the back or the muscles and ligaments that cross the back of the knee joint, some authorities recommend avoiding this exercise in favor of sitting toe touches. If one chooses to "bounce," these should be done gently (see Concept 7 on Flexibility). (171, 234, 235)

6. Rising on the Toes and Heels—The "tiptoeing" exercise will develop the calf muscles, but at the same time it stretches the muscles and ligaments that help support the long arch of the foot. "Heel-walking" may have the same effect—that is, develop already strong muscles while the arch of the foot is further weakened. The potential harm is lessened if these exercises are performed with the toes turned in slightly. (2, 185)

7. Isometric Exercises—As previously pointed out, this type of exercise develops strength but does not contribute to cardiovascular fitness or flexibility. One study has shown such a program to be more dangerous to heart patients than isotonic exercises, since twice as many patients developed irregular heart beats during isometric testing than they did on the bicycle exerciser. (2)

8. "Slimming Wheels"—This popular device is a small wheel with a handle passing through its center. It is used in a push-up type exercise, advertised for back and abdominal strengthening. Little research has been done to prove its value, but one hospital has reported a case of abdominal muscle hemorrhaging resulting from the use of the wheel. (2) One should not strive for that "familiar soreness" in the exercise

of the abdominals, but rather should discontinue exercise when a feeling of discomfort occurs. (181)

Exercise, even of an active nature, is NOT effective in promoting physical fitness unless the exercise meets the appropriate threshold of training.

Recent popular literature suggests that only a few minutes of exercise a day is necessary to develop total physical fitness. (201) Research evidence indicates that total fitness (cardiovascular fitness, strength, muscular endurance, flexibility, and desirable body composition) can be attained only through considerable effort. As mentioned previously in this text, exercise must be of sufficient intensity, frequency (daily or every other day), and duration (at least fifteen to thirty minutes *each day* you exercise) if it is to be effective. Programs "promising" complete fitness that do not meet the necessary levels for intensity, frequency, and duration of exercise should be strongly questioned.

Sauna, steam, and whirlpool baths are NOT effective in weight reduction nor in the prevention and cure of colds, arthritis, bursitis, backaches, sprains, and bruises.

The effect of such baths is largely psychological, although some temporary relief from aches and pains may result from the heat. The same effect can be had by sitting in a tub of hot water at home. (182) Sauna and steam baths are potentially dangerous for the elderly and persons suffering from diabetes, heart disease, or high blood pressure. They should not be used within an hour of eating or while under the influence of alcohol or drugs such as anticoagulants, stimulants, hypnotics, narcotics, or tranquilizers. (96)

Health clubs and/or reducing salons may lack qualified personnel for advising or prescribing exercise programs or diets. (180, 258)

Studies indicate that the majority of the salons or clubs lack personnel with special training or education in such recognized fields as physical therapy, corrective therapy, or physical education. The employees had not taken such courses as anatomy, physiology, kinesiology, exercise therapy, or nutrition. Most of their training had consisted of two or three weeks of on-the-job experience.

Exercise tests are necessary to determine physical fitness, but certain cautions should be observed.

No exercise program should be undertaken without the approval of a physician. Sedentary individuals need a thorough physical exam and a stress test to detect ischemic heart disease and to evaluate cardiac fitness. These tests should be administered by trained individuals with resuscitation equipment easily available, but the risk is very low in normal subjects [no greater than a number of medical procedures such as coronary angiography]. (232, 240, 257)

Jogging is an excellent exercise for cardiovascular conditioning, weight control, and improvement of a variety of conditions; however, reasonable cautions should be observed. (58, 114, 176, 188, 115)

Jogging has been used successfully in the rehabilitation of cardiac patients and pulmonary emphysema; reducing diabetics; relaxing insomniacs, emotionally disturbed, and migraine patients; incontinence after pregnancy; and arthritis in legs and back. A regular program will decrease the risk of coronary artery disease. Specific guidelines for post-coronary joggers have been outlined recently. (152)

Jogging should not be undertaken without a physician's approval, especially for those with osteoporosis and heart and circulatory diseases. Contrary to the opinion of some detractors (241), *there is no evidence* that jogging will cause low back pain, hernias, varicose veins, phlebitis, or uterus and breast problems. If some of these problems already exist, jogging might aggravate the condition. (174)

Jogging *can cause* shin splints, blisters, and foot, ankle, and hip problems. Proper footwear and learning how to jog properly will minimize these hazards.

Dehydration, a hazard in certain sports and exercise situations, is a serious medical problem.

Excessive loss of body fluids and an accompanying loss of electrolytes can impair performance and lead to illness or even death. Weight losing gimmicks (including high protein-low carbohydrate diets) that cause dehydration are dangerous, especially for athletes (e.g., wrestlers trying to "make weight").

Athletes subjected to heat stress should weigh before and after practice and replace water loss; water intake should *not* be restricted during practice. It is doubtful that any beneficial effects accrue from adding electrolytes to water ingested after dehydration. The person regularly exposed to vigorous physical activity with heat stress may benefit from drinking a quart of milk and two eight-ounce glasses of orange juice per day. (52, 67, 174, 147)

The hazards of drugs far outweigh any improvement in athletic performance that might result from their use.

Authorities disagree on whether drugs can enhance athletic performance. Examples of research studies include evidence that suggests increased intake of vitamin E does not improve endurance. (176) Anabolic steroids have been shown to temporarily increase strength when combined with a high protein diet and exercise, but the serious side effects make them inadvisable. (103) "Doping" of athletes has included the use of drugs ranging from caffeine and vitamins to cocaine, strychnine, adrenalin, tranquilizers, and narcotics.

Drugs can make a person feel like he/she has performed well whether he/she has or not; they also tend to mask symptoms that are important in knowing when the body is being taxed beyond safe limits; almost all drugs have side effects and these can sometimes be dangerous; drugs can be addictive. When sports are conducted on the basis of pharmacological expertise rather than on athletic competence, the traditional philosophy and spirit of competition is lost. (55, 164)

There are certain hazards inherent in exercise that should be minimized by proper technique, knowledgeable instructors, proper equipment and apparel, and judicious practice schedules.

Some examples of exercise hazards are included here.

Weight-lifters may be subject to inguinal hernias and blackouts as a result of the Valsalva maneuver. This can be prevented by avoiding hyperventilation, squatting as briefly as possible, and raising the weight as rapidly as possible to a position in which it can be supported while normal breathing is resumed. (50)

Excess activity during the adolescent stage may result in a degeneration of the hip joint and knee joints, especially among boys, and especially in the presence of growing pains. (204) This suggests parents and coaches should examine all the evidence related to athletics during this so-called "dangerous age." The merit of long-distance runs, particularly on hard surfaces, as a form of athletic training should also be examined.

Most runners and occasionally joggers at some time complain of "shin splints." This usually disappears within a few weeks and often can be prevented by proper technique, but one form of the injury may require surgery. For most individuals the exercises presented in this text will be of benefit, however, if pain persists or is unusually severe, a physician should be consulted. (221)

Suggested Readings

Cooper, D. "Drugs and the Athlete," *Journal of the American Medical Association* 221 (August 28, 1972):107.

Kuntzleman, C. "Dangerous Exercises: Which, When, Why," *Fitness for Living,* January-February, 1971, pp. 25-29.

Lamb, L. E. "Playboy's Jogging Prank," *Health Newsletter* VII (June 11, 1976): 11.

"What You Should Know Before Joining a Health Club," *Today's Health,* February, 1971, p. 17.

In order to attain maximal benefits from exercise it is essential that a regular progressive program be planned to meet the specific needs of the individual.

Planning Your Exercise Program

Concept 19

In order to attain maximal benefits from exercise it is essential that a regular progressive program be planned to meet the specific needs of the individual.

Introduction

Every individual has unique physical fitness needs. Prior to planning a program of physical fitness the following factors should be considered:

1. The program should be based on an evaluation of the individual's present fitness status.
2. Fitness cannot be developed overnight. The exercise program should progress from moderate to more vigorous exercises until the desired fitness level is attained.
3. The program should be regular. This means at *least* three times a week.
4. Every aspect of fitness should be considered in developing a physical fitness program.
5. An exercise program should do more than *just* develop physical fitness. Plan a program you enjoy.

The Facts

The first step in planning an exercise program is IDENTIFYING YOUR INDIVIDUAL NEEDS.

Before you begin an exercise program you should identify your exercise needs, a process that involves two basic steps: GETTING A MEDICAL EXAMINATION and TESTING YOURSELF FOR EACH ASPECT OF PHYSICAL FITNESS. Information concerning fitness self-testing and standards for rating your physical fitness are presented in Labs 5, 6, 7 (cardiovascular fitness); 8, 9 (strength); 10 (muscular endurance); 11 (flexibility); 12, 13 (fatness); 21, 22 (posture and back care); 15, 16, 17, 18 (skill-related fitness); and 19, 20 (body mechanics).

The second step in planning an exercise program is LEARNING WHICH EXERCISES DO WHAT.

Exercise is an excellent way to achieve fitness and one means of attaining good health. However, all exercise is not necessarily good. Once you know what your exercise needs are make sure you are aware of the facts about exercise.

BE SURE THE EXERCISES YOU SELECT MEET THE NEEDS THAT *YOU* HAVE AND MAKE SURE THAT THE EXERCISES YOU SELECT MEET THE THRESHOLD OF TRAINING FOR YOU. Information concerning the facts about exercise and the threshold of training for each aspect of fitness are presented in the preceding sections of this book. Labs 25 to 37 and Appendixes A^1 to A^{14} present samples of various types of exercises and discuss the strengths and weaknesses of each.

The third step in planning an exercise program is MAKING SURE THAT YOU ARE MEETING ALL OF YOUR EXERCISE NEEDS.

Once you have determined what your exercise needs are and which exercises do what, it is important to make sure that you are exercising to meet all of your exercise needs. NO SINGLE EXERCISE CAN MEET ALL OF YOUR NEEDS. Make sure you have selected exercises for all aspects of physical fitness and especially MAKE SURE THAT YOU HAVE SELECTED A PROGRAM THAT YOU ENJOY. THE BEST PROGRAM IN THE WORLD IS NOT GOOD UNLESS YOU DO IT. If you don't enjoy it, you may not do it.

The fourth step in planning an exercise program is to WRITE IT DOWN.

You are more likely to do your exercise program if you write it down. Lab 38 provides a place to record your exercise program.

The final step in planning the program is to SELECT A REGULAR TIME AND PLACE FOR YOUR EXERCISE.

Regularity is one of the keys to the success of your exercise program. The "hit or miss" program is likely to evolve into no program at all. From the beginning set a time and a place for your activity. Place a high priority on your exercise time. DON'T ALLOW JUST ANYTHING TO INTERRUPT YOUR EXERCISE. Build your exercise program into your daily routine; make it as much a habit as taking a bath or eating regular meals. It is recommended that some form of exercise be done daily; three days a week should be a minimum.

There are some important GUIDELINES for carrying out the well-planned exercise program.

1. *An exercise program should be started gradually to avoid soreness or injury.* (181) Begin with a minimum of repetitions (or load) and gradually increase them over a period of time. If anything, "underexercise" rather than "overexercise" initially. Some muscle soreness can be expected if you are unaccustomed to activity, but repeating the exercises the next day will alleviate it. Much soreness and possible strain can be avoided by progressing gradually, by warming-up with a few mild stretching and circulatory exercises, and by performing the exercises slowly and deliberately with no quick jerky movements. To avoid injury to the abdominals, start slow, avoid soreness in the area and do not hold your breath during exertion. Breathe normally or try to inhale during the recovery phase and exhale during the effort phase of an exercise.

2. *Periodically vary your exercise program.* Repeating the same program over a long period of time may result in loss of interest. Since there are many different types of physical activity that can result in similar types of fitness improvement, consider changing your program from time to time.

3. *Avoid those exercises that are termed "questionable."* Certain exercises have dangers to the typical person and may result in injury. These exercises should be avoided (see Concept 18). Also be sure to exercise through the full range of joint movement. Do not hurry through your exercises, especially weight training and calisthenics.

4. *Make exercise fun.* Wear appropriate clothing and keep the exercise period short and well organized. To make the session more interesting and provide more motivation, exercise with a partner or a group. To help break the monotony of a routine, vary the program by changing exercises and by performing to musical accompaniment or while watching T.V. When doing calisthenics on the floor, use padding to avoid pressure on bony areas that might become bruised.

5. *Set realistic goals and measure your progress.* (181) Set goals that you have a reasonable chance to attain and do not expect miracles. Since you did not become "unfit" overnight, do not expect to become "fit" in a day. It is a slow process, but periodical reevaluation will boost your morale by revealing progress. When your initial goals are met, you may wish to set higher goals. Some of the same tests for assessing your exercise needs can be used to measure your progress.

6. *Warm-up and cool-down before and after moderate to vigorous physical activity.* Recent research indicates that in addition to warming up the skeletal muscles before exercise, the heart muscle should be warmed up. Research results indicate that approximately two minutes of easy jogging should precede moderate to vigorous activity to im-

prove blood flow to the heart. This is necessary since, for many adults, blood flow to the heart does not increase instantly at the beginning of work by the heart. (12)

There are those who believe that a warm-up is also advised for the skeletal muscles. Those who hold this position feel that passive stretching of the muscles prior to moderate or vigorous exercise can reduce muscle soreness and possible muscle injury. Others, most notably Dr. A. J. Ryan, feel that similar stretching exercises may be beneficial after activity as well. (127)

"Cooling down" or tapering off after exercise is also important. After moderate to vigorous activity it is wise to gradually decrease the amount of activity performed as opposed to stopping abruptly. After a jog or a bout of exercise, you should continue to walk and move around, particularly the legs should continue to move.

During exercise much blood is pumped to the large muscles of the legs. If you stop exercising abruptly much of the blood pumped to the leg muscles is left there with no quick way provided for that blood to return to the heart. If you walk around, the massaging action of the muscles will move the blood out of the legs and back to the heart. If too much blood is pumped to the legs and not back to the heart muscle it could cause a person to "pass out" after exercise.

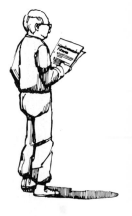

Physical activity and exercise can contribute to physical fitness, good health, and an improved quality of life for people of all ages.

Exercise for a Lifetime

Concept 20

Physical activity and exercise can contribute to physical fitness, good health, and an improved quality of life for people of all ages.

Introduction

In our culture activity is often for the older child, the adolescent, and the young adult. Yet research evidence indicates that *all people* including young children and older people can benefit from regular physical activity.

Terms

Acquired aging—The acquisition of characteristics commonly associated with aging but that are in fact caused by immobility or inactivity.

Time dependent aging—The loss of function resulting from growing older.

The Facts

Physical Activity for Children

Children, even very young children, are quite capable of vigorous physical activity. However, the optimal time for development of high levels of health-related fitness occurs after the beginning of adolescence.

Children can exercise regularly. The typical child needs several hours of large muscle activity daily. For their body size children can perform equal to young adults, but should not (because of their smaller size and because they are not mature emotionally) be expected to compete with adolescents and young adults. (65)

A healthy child cannot physiologically injure his or her heart through physical exercise. (62)

Parents should not be concerned about the old wives' tale that suggests that exercise for children will result in damage to the heart. Research

...s this myth. At the same time, children are not miniature adults
...d programs of exercise for health-related fitness, including cardiovascular fitness, should be designed to meet both the physical and psychological needs and interests of children. Too much too soon may breed dislike for any type of physical activity.

Children should be exposed to a wide variety of physical activity experiences in order to establish a basis for a lifetime of activity. (62)

Recent research indicates that nearly all Americans have had some physical education during their school years. Nevertheless, only 40 percent of all school children have physical education in the elementary school. (220) Evidence indicates that most skills are learned by age twelve or by the end of the sixth grade. (205) For this reason, it is important that children not specialize in one activity too early thus allowing more time to concentrate on learning as many activities as possible during the school years. Just as a child learning to read must first learn the alphabet and grammar, the child in physical activity should be exposed to many fundamental activities early in life so that he or she can take advantage of more than one lifetime activity in adulthood.

Physical Activity for the Adolescent

It is during adolescence that exercise contributes the most dramatic improvements in health-related physical fitness. (78)

During adolescence hormonal changes occur that promote dramatic increases in cardiovascular fitness and strength with regular exercise. Both boys and girls can improve significantly in fitness at this age with regular exercise.

Adolescence is a time when the social aspects of sports competition and participation can provide great satisfaction to both the participant and the spectator.

Because adolescence is a social age and because sports and sporting events provide social experiences, sports can be a significant part of the life of the adolescent. However, for a lifetime of exercise the adolescent should be encouraged to become involved in sport as a participant as opposed to becoming only a spectator.

Adolescence is a good time to refine lifetime sports skills.

Though most skills are learned early in life it is during adolescence that lifetime sports skills are refined. Adolescents acquire the health-related, as well as the skill-related, fitness necessary to refine and become efficient in sports skills. Adolescents should be exposed to a variety of skills that can be used for a lifetime.

Physical Activity for Adults (Age 17 Plus)

Most of the limitations of adults in exercise are self-imposed. (78)

Approximately 49 million of 109 million adult American men and women do not engage in physical activity for the purpose of exercise (220). Of those who do not exercise regularly it is their own lack of fitness resulting from years of inactivity that makes them feel unable to participate. While one of five American adults has been told by a physician to exercise, rarely does a physician suggest inactivity except for short periods of time for a specific ailment.

The "weekend" adult athlete may create rather than solve exercise problems.

A "weekend athlete" is one who exercises, sometimes vigorously, only on the weekend. This person may avoid exercise during the "busy" weekdays and attempt to "make up" for a week of inactivity on Saturday or Sunday. To be effective, exercise must be regular (at least three times a week). Vigorous exercise done only one day a week can be dangerous because the weekly exercise is not sufficient to produce improvements in fitness. Thus the unfit person may be exposing himself or herself to exercise for which the body is not prepared.

Being "TOO BUSY" is not a good excuse for inactivity.

The most common reason for inactivity among adults is, "I can't take the time." If business or other obligations make it such that weekday activities in golf or tennis are impossible then walking, jogging, or calisthenics are appropriate. These activities take relatively little time and if planned properly can provide important fitness and health benefits. After the inactive person has had a heart attack or some other hypokinetic disease, he or she will have more free time than they really want. Exercise may be as important as food and, like meals, should be scheduled every day.

Physical Activity for Older Adults

Adults are never "too old" to begin exercising. (80)

Physical fitness for old age should begin in the early years in order for maximum benefits to come to each individual. If this does not occur for one reason or another, one is never too old to begin exercising. (80) Studies conducted over a period of years indicate that properly planned exercise for older people is not only safe but that older men and women are NOT significantly different from youth (in a relative sense) when it comes to improving fitness through exercise. (80)

Regular exercise can have a significant delaying effect on the aging process. (80, 89, 175)

One researcher suggests that "exercise is the closest thing to an antiaging pill now available." (36, p. 67) Another indicates that continued mental and physical activity is ". . . the only antidote for aging that I know." (162, p. 93)

There is a difference between "acquired aging" and "time-dependent aging." (175)

Forced inactivity in young adults has been shown to cause losses in function (acquired aging) that are very much like those that we generally consider to occur with aging (time-dependent aging). Recent studies conducted on older adults over a long period of time suggest that aging appears to be more a product of a sedentary life-style than of aging. (223) Studies in Africa, Asia, and South America, where older adults (age 65 and older) maintain an active life-style, show that these individuals do not "acquire" many of the characteristics commonly associated with aging. (89)

In our culture middle-aged and older people are encouraged (and sometimes compelled) to reduce their physical activity to the extent that they cannot continue to function on their own. (161)

In our society the attitude toward older people is often one of overprotection, placing the person in a position of being dependent. A spokesperson for the President's Council for Physical Fitness and Sports suggests that ". . . a state of physical fitness enhances the quality of life for the elderly by increasing independence. The ability to 'go places and do things' without being dependent on others provides a strong psychological lift which is conducive to good mental health." (51, p. 83)

Participation in regular activity has benefits other than improved physical health and fitness.

A general feeling of "well-being" is frequently reported to be one of the real benefits of regular fitness for older people. Nervous tension, which detracts from the feeling of well-being, is a problem of many older adults. One recent study showed that exercise can be more effective than tranquilizers in the treatment of nervous tension in older people. (80)

Participation in regular physical activity has many physical health benefits for the older adult.

In addition to the health benefits of exercise already presented in this book, there are other benefits to older adults that result from regular physical activity.

1. "The syndrome of shaky hand and tottery gait is responsible in a large degree for much of the dependency of the aged. The treatment (of this condition) is physical exercise." (264, p. 7) Merely fifteen minutes of exercise a day will not do it, rather there must be a shift from a sedentary to an active life-style.

2. Studies at Duke University Center for the Study of Aging indicate that active older people have fewer illnesses and fewer early deaths than do those who are inactive. (223)

3. Studies show that reductions in physical working capacity, which is the most obvious result of aging, do not occur in older men who engage in regular exercise. Researchers indicate that regular exercise prevents the expected decline in physical working capacity. (150)

4. Regular exercise can help older adults in the "War with Gravity." Gravity has its effect on the human body. With time, if muscles are not kept fit, gravity can cause "Bay Window" or protruding abdomen, sagging shoulders, poor posture, and joint immobility. All of these "gravity" problems result from lack of strength, muscular endurance, and flexibility and can be forestalled with regular activity. (175)

5. Bones that are not used tend to decalcify. Regular exercise for older adults can delay decalcification of bones. (175)

6. With age the ability of the heart to function effectively as a pump decreases for the typical adult. This decrease is at the rate of 1 percent per year after adulthood. Regular exercise can forestall the decline in circulatory function. In addition normal increases in atherosclerosis, blood pressure, and EKG abnormalities that occur with age can be prevented with appropriate regular exercise. (80)

7. Other changes in function that occur in "normal" adults with age include decreased skeletal muscle, gain in body fat, decrease in oxygen use capacity, and decreased respiratory function. These changes in function can be postponed with regular exercise. (73, 80)

Older adults can participate in a wide variety of sports and physical activity.

Older adults have shown that with appropriate progressively maintained exercise they can participate in most sports for a lifetime. For example one man of age eighty-five regularly plays handball (161) and the increased participation in masters (over 50) classifications in track and field, swimming, and tennis are well documented. Bowling is the leading participant sport in the United States and is well suited for older people. Golf is another activity well suited for older Americans. For those who do not wish to choose a sport, walking, jogging, bicycle riding, swimming, and calisthenics are forms of physical activity that are widely used by people of all ages.

Older adults should be especially careful to follow the exercise guidelines presented in Concept 19.

Suggested Readings

"Testimony on Physical Fitness for Older Persons." Washington, D. C.: National Association for Human Development, 1975. Reprinted and available from the President's Council on Physical Fitness and Sports, Washington, D. C. 20201.

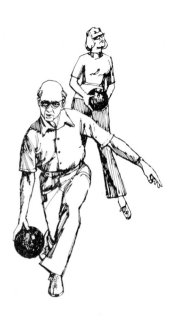

The Values of Physical Activity

Name_____ Section_____ Date_____

Purpose

The purpose of this laboratory session is to evaluate individual attitudes about the value of physical activity.

Procedures

Read each of the sixteen items listed on page 137 and answer them "strongly agree," "agree," "undecided," "disagree," or "strongly disagree." Give the one answer that best indicates the way YOU feel. Try not to use the response "undecided" unless absolutely necessary. Score the sixteen items using the scoring method on page 138.

Expected Results

People participate in sports, physical activity, and exercise for different reasons. For which reason do you think you choose to exercise or choose not to exercise? Check the box or boxes that apply to you.

I exercise for physical fitness. ☐
I exercise for social reasons. ☐
I exercise to relax. ☐
I exercise because I think I should. ☐
If other reasons—list them here:

I do not choose to exercise regularly. ☐

Results

The sixteen-item test is designed to help you determine your attitude toward physical activity. There are different reasons for participation, and your scores will help you to better understand your reasons for choosing to exercise or not to exercise. How did you score on each of the scales?

	Ex.	Good	N	Poor	VP
Health and Physical Fitness	☐	☐	☐	☐	☐
Social	☐	☐	☐	☐	☐
Recreation-Relaxation	☐	☐	☐	☐	☐
General	☐	☐	☐	☐	☐

Conclusions

Did you score as you expected? Yes ☐ No ☐
Why or why not?

Implications

Of what significance is your attitude toward physical education with reference to your future participation in sports and activity? Could anything be done to change your attitude? When did you establish your basic attitude toward activity, sports, and exercise?

Read each of the statements listed below and check the box that best represents your feeling about the statement.

Attitude Test

Strongly Agree	Agree	Unde-cided	Dis-agree	Strongly Disagree		SCORE
☐	☐	☐	☐	☑	1. Physical education is all right for those who like sports but is not for me.	_____
☐	☐	☐	☐	☐	2. Physical exercise and activity are as dangerous to health as they are valuable.	_____
☐	☐	☐	☐	☐	3. I enjoy taking part in a sport just to get away from it all.	_____
☐	☐	☐	☐	☐	4. I like to participate best in those games that involve working as a team.	_____
☐	☐	☐	☐	☐	5. Physical activity is one way to rid yourself of the worries and tensions of everyday life.	_____
☐	☐	☐	☐	☐	6. Probably one of the main values of sports is to fill leisure time in our automated society.	_____
☐	☐	☐	☐	☐	7. I would only enroll in physical education if it were a graduation requirement.	_____
☐	☐	☐	☐	☐	8. The time some people spend exercising could probably be better spent in other ways.	_____
☐	☐	☐	☐	☐	9. Sports and games build social confidence.	_____
☐	☐	☐	☐	☐	10. Industry might be wise to substitute exercise breaks for coffee breaks.	_____
☐	☐	☐	☐	☐	11. Competition in sports is often a way to destroy good friendships.	_____
☐	☐	☐	☐	☐	12. Most jobs provide all the exercise and activity a person needs.	_____
☐	☐	☐	☐	☐	13. Everyone should have skill in several sports that can be used later in life.	_____
☐	☐	☐	☐	☐	14. Social dancing and other similar forms of activity are a waste of time.	_____
☐	☐	☐	☐	☐	15. Health and physical fitness are basic to all of life's activities.	_____
☐	☐	☐	☐	☐	16. I would recommend that everyone take physical education because of the important nature of the subject.	_____

Score the attitude test as follows:

1. For items 1, 2, 7, 8, 11, 12, and 14 give one point for Strongly Agree, two for Agree, three for Undecided, four for Disagree, and five for Strongly disagree. Put the correct number on the blank to the right of these statements.
2. For items 3, 4, 5, 6, 9, 10, 13, 15, and 16 give five points for Strongly Agree, four for Agree, three for Undecided, two for Disagree, and one for Strongly Disagree. Put the correct number on the blank to the right of these statements.
3. Add the scores for items 2, 8, 12, and 15. This total represents your health and fitness attitude score.
4. Add the scores for items 4, 9, 11, and 14. This total represents your social attitude score.
5. Add the scores for items 3, 5, 6, and 13. This total represents your recreational-emotional attitude score.
6. Add the scores for items 1, 7, 10, and 16. This total represents your general attitude score.
7. Circle your scores on the chart given and record them on page 135.

Attitude Rating Scale

	Attitude Scale First Test				
	HF Scale	Social	Rec-Emot	General	Total
Excellent (Ex)	18	18	18	18	69-72
Good	15-17	15-17	15-17	15-17	57-68
Marginal (M)	8-14	8-14	8-14	8-14	32-56
Poor	6-7	6-7	6-7	6-7	21-31
Very Poor (VP)	0-5	0-5	0-5	0-5	0-20

8. Record your results by circling the appropriate score above. Determine your rating for each scale and record it in the results section.

Exercise and the Heart

Name _____ Section _____ Date _____

Purpose

The purposes of this laboratory session are:

1. To discover which physical activities allow the heart to slow down and rest.
2. To discover which physical activities cause greatest overload on the heart muscle.
3. To discover which physical activities allow the quickest and most efficient recovery from exercise overload.

Procedures

1. Practice taking your carotid pulse for several thirty-second periods. The instructor will show you how and will signal by saying "Start" and "Stop" before and after several thirty-second periods at rest.
2. Take your thirty-second pulse after each of the following:
   a. standing at attention for one minute
   b. performing three minutes of a vigorous exercise of your choice (running, sit-ups, rope jumping, etc.)
   c. one minute of recovery from the exercise above (take a sitting position to aid the heart in returning to normal)
   d. two minutes of recovery from the exercise above
   e. three minutes of recovery from the exercise above
   f. four minutes of recovery from the exercise above
3. Record results on the graph in the results section.

Expected Results

What is your "threshold of training"? _____ Beats per min.

How high do you expect your heart rate to go after three minutes of exercise? _____ Beats per min.

How long do you think it will take for your heart rate to return to normal? _____

Results

Record heart rates for activities on the following bar graph.
Darken the appropriate bar to the proper level.

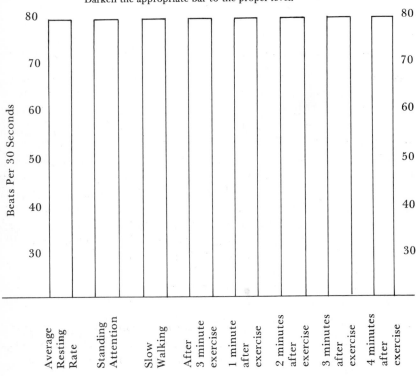

Conclusions

Did your heart rate return to normal at any time after the beginning of
the lab session? Yes ☐ No ☐

Implications

What practical implications can you draw from this experiment?

The Cardiovascular Threshold of Training

Name_____ Section_____ Date_____

Minimal amounts of exercise will not produce increases in cardiovascular fitness. Researchers suggest that exercise must be vigorous enough to elevate the heart rate to a "minimum threshold" value if the exercise is to be effective in producing fitness. The minimum threshold is considerably above the resting heart rate but varies from individual to individual depending on each person's resting heart rate, age, and maximal heart rate. Chart 4.1 presents the "threshold of training" values for different individuals based on age and resting heart rate. Since maximal heart rate is very difficult to determine, the typical maximal heart rate for each age group was used in preparing the chart. The heart rate should be held at the level of the "threshold of training" for a minimum of ten to fifteen minutes if exercise is to be effective.

Purpose

The purpose of this laboratory session is to help you discover how much exercise is necessary to elevate the heart rate to threshold level. More specifically the purpose of the lab session is to help each individual:

1. Understand the "threshold of training" concept.
2. Establish a personal minimal cardiovascular "threshold of training."
3. Determine the specific speed of jogging necessary to elevate the heart rate to "threshold of training" level.

Procedures

1. Find your threshold of training on Chart 4.1, page 147.
2. Select a partner.
3. One partner should run a quarter mile, the other partner should count her or his (use carotid pulse) heart rate at the end of the run. Try to run at a rate that you think will keep the rate of the heart in the threshold of training.
4. Repeat, alternating roles, one running, one counting heart rate.
5. Repeat the test so each person runs twice.
6. Record heart rates in the "results" section of this experiment.

Results

What is your "threshold of training" (from Chart 4.1)? _____ BPM
What was your heart rate for the first run? _____ BPM
What was your heart rate for the second run? _____ BPM

Conclusions

How fast would you need to run a mile to achieve your cardiovascular
threshold of training as noted in Chart 4.1? _____
Could you do it? Yes ☐ No ☐

Implications

Does the average American achieve the cardiovascular threshold of training in the course of a normal day? Yes ☐ No ☐
What would you suggest for yourself as a regular daily cardiovascular exercise program?

Minimum Heart Rates necessary to produce improved cardiovascular fitness.

Resting Heart Rate	Experience**	Age									
		less than 25	25-29	30-34	35-39	40-44	45-49	50-54	55-59	60-64	over 65
below 45	Beginner	134-138	131-135	128-132	125-129	122-126	119-123	116-120	113-117	110-114	107-111
	Experienced	149-153	145-149	142-146	139-143	136-140	132-136	129-133	125-129	122-126	118-122
45-49	Beginner	136-140	133-137	130-134	127-131	124-128	121-125	118-122	115-119	112-116	109-113
	Experienced	151-155	147-151	144-148	141-145	137-141	134-138	130-134	127-131	123-127	120-124
50-54	Beginner	138-142	135-139	132-136	129-133	126-130	123-127	120-124	117-121	114-118	111-115
	Experienced	153-157	149-153	145-149	142-146	139-143	135-139	132-136	128-132	125-129	121-125
55-59	Beginner	140-144	137-141	134-138	131-135	128-132	125-129	122-126	119-123	116-120	113-117
	Experienced	154-158	150-154	147-151	144-148	140-144	137-141	133-137	130-134	126-130	123-127
60-64	Beginner	142-146	139-143	136-140	133-137	130-134	127-131	124-128	121-125	118-122	115-119
	Experienced	156-160	152-156	149-153	145-149	142-146	138-142	135-139	131-135	128-132	124-128
65-69	Beginner	144-148	141-145	138-142	135-139	132-136	129-133	126-130	123-127	120-124	117-121
	Experienced	157-161	154-158	150-154	146-150	143-147	140-144	136-140	133-137	129-133	126-130
70-74	Beginner	146-150	143-147	140-144	137-141	134-138	131-135	128-132	125-129	122-126	119-123
	Experienced	158-162	155-159	152-156	148-150	145-149	141-145	138-142	134-138	131-135	127-131
75-79	Beginner	146-150	145-149	142-146	139-143	136-140	133-137	130-134	127-131	124-128	121-125
	Experienced	158-162	157-161	154-158	149-153	146-150	143-147	139-143	136-140	132-136	129-133
80 and over	Beginner	146-150	145-149	144-148	141-145	138-142	135-141	132-136	129-133	126-130	123-127
	Experienced	158-162	157-161	155-160	151-155	148-152	144-148	141-145	137-141	134-138	130-134

*Based on Maximal Heart Rates suggested by Astrand (9) and Modification of the Threshold of Training Formula suggested by Karvonen (149).

***Beginners* are individuals just starting exercise for the first time or beginning again after more than a four-week layoff. *Experienced* are individuals who have participated in a regular exercise program for at least six weeks duration.

Evaluating Cardiovascular Fitness– The Twelve-Minute Run

Name _____ Section _____ Date _____

When you engage in a regular exercise program you need some type of evaluation to determine your progress. One of the best methods of evaluating cardiovascular fitness is a test called Maximal Oxygen Uptake. It is an all-out test that takes several hours to complete. A more practical test is the Twelve-Minute Run, which requires very little equipment. The Twelve-Minute Run test was developed by Dr. Kenneth Cooper (56) and is considered to be better than runs of other lengths for assessing cardiovascular fitness.

Purpose

The purpose of this laboratory session is to evaluate your cardiovascular fitness and to acquaint you with an effective means of evaluating cardiovascular fitness throughout life.

Procedures

Perform the Twelve-Minute Run and record your score in the result section of this report. To perform the test you should run as far as possible during a twelve-minute period. The further the distance the better the score. Attempt to establish a steady pace that can be maintained for the full twelve-minute period.

Expected Results

Check the classification you expect to achieve on this test of cardiovascular fitness. Excellent ☐ Very good ☐ Marginal ☐ Poor ☐ Very poor ☐
How far do you expect to run on this test? _____

Results

What distance did you cover in twelve minutes? _____
What is your rating? _____ (See Rating Scale on page 151).

Conclusions and Implications

Did you score as well as you thought you would? Yes ☐ No ☐
Did you score better than you thought? Yes ☐ No ☐
Does this test indicate your true fitness level? Yes ☐ No ☐
What do the results of this test imply to you about your exercise needs?

Use the following table to determine your rating on the twelve-minute run. The table is for persons seventeen to twenty-five years of age. Older persons should use the tables for older adults.

Table 5.1

Classification	Men	Women
Excellent	1.9 miles	1.5 miles
Very Good	1.8-1.89 miles	1.4-1.49 miles
Marginal	1.6-1.79 miles	1.1-1.39 miles
Poor	1.5-1.59 miles	1.0-1.09 miles
Very Poor	1.4-1.49 miles	below .9 miles

The following tables are provided to help you evaluate your fitness as you get older. You may wish to make these charts available to an older friend or relative.

Table 5.2 Twelve-Minute Test for Men*

(Distances in miles covered in twelve minutes)

Fitness Category	26–39	40–49	50+
I. Very Poor	<.95	<.85	<.80
II. Poor	.95–1.14	.85–1.04	.80– .99
III. Fair	1.15–1.39	1.05–1.29	1.0 –1.24
IV. Good	1.40–1.64	1.30–1.54	1.25–1.49
V. Excellent	1.65+	1.55+	1.50+

Twelve-Minute Test for Women*

(Distances in miles covered in twelve minutes)

Fitness Category	26–39	40–49	50+
I. Very Poor	<.85	<.75	<.65
II. Poor	.85–1.04	.75– .94	.65– .84
III. Fair	1.05–1.24	.95–1.14	.85–1.04
IV. Good	1.25–1.54	1.15–1.44	1.05–1.34
V. Excellent	1.55+	1.45+	1.35+

*Adapted from Cooper (58).

Evaluating Cardiovascular Fitness–
The Step Test

Lab **6**

Name_____ Section_____ Date_____

When you engage in a regular exercise program you need some type of evaluation to determine your progress. Laboratory 5 explains one practical test for measuring cardiovascular fitness—the "Twelve-Minute Run." This lab explains "The Step Test," another practical test that requires very little equipment. There are several modifications of the "Step Test." The Kasch Three-Minute Step Test* is used for this laboratory session because it can be performed by all age groups and by both sexes. Only extremely unfit or ill persons would find the test too strenuous.

Purpose

The purpose of this laboratory session is to evaluate your cardiovascular fitness and to acquaint you with an effective means of evaluating cardiovascular fitness throughout life.

Procedure

1. Choose a partner. After you exercise, your partner will count your pulse.
2. Step up and down on a twelve-inch bench for three minutes at a rate of twenty-four steps a minute.**
3. Immediately after exercise sit down on the bench and relax. Don't talk.
4. Your partner will locate your carotid pulse. Five seconds after exercise your partner will count your pulse for sixty seconds.
5. Your score is the sixty-second pulse rate. Find your score in Chart 6.1 to determine your cardiovascular fitness rating.
6. Record your rating in the results section of the lab.
7. Now count for your partner after he/she does three minutes of stepping.

*Adapted from Kasch, F. W. and Boyer, J. L. *Adult Fitness: Principles and Practices*. Palo Alto, Calif.: Mayfield Publishers, 1968.
**"One step" consists of: up with the right foot, up with the left foot, down with the right foot, and down with the left foot. Completely straighten the legs as you step up on the bench.

The Step Test

153

Expected Results

How do you expect to
perform on the Step Test?

Results

What was your heart rate
at the end of the test?
What was your rating
(see Chart 6.1)?

Excellent	☐
Very Good	☐
Marginal	☐
Poor	☐
Very Poor	☐

Excellent	☐
Very Good	☐
Marginal	☐
Poor	☐
Very Poor	☐

Conclusions and Implications

Did you score as well as you thought you would? Yes ☐ No ☐
Did you score better than you thought you would? Yes ☐ No ☐
Do you think this test is a true measure of your cardiovascular fitness?
Yes ☐ No ☐
What do the results of this test imply to your need for exercise?

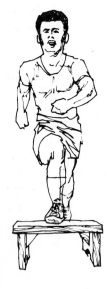

Chart 6.1 Step Test Rating Chart*

Classification	Sixty-second Heart Rate
Excellent	80 or less
Very Good	81- 90
Marginal	91-110
Poor	111-120
Very Poor	121 and above

*As you grow older you would want to continue to score well
on this rating chart. Because your maximal heart rate decreases as you grow older you should be able to score well if
you exercise regularly.

Evaluating Cardiovascular Fitness– The Astrand-Ryhming Bicycle Test

Name_____Section_____Date_____

When you engage in a regular exercise program you need some type of evaluation to determine your progress. The Step Test and the Twelve-Minute Run are good substitutes for the more scientific Maximal Oxygen Uptake Test because they require very little equipment. However, if the equipment is available the Astrand-Ryhming Bicycle Test is probably a better substitute predictor of Maximal Oxygen Uptake than either of the tests used in Labs 5 or 6.

Purpose

The purpose of this laboratory session is to evaluate the individual's cardiovascular fitness and to acquaint the student with an effective means of evaluating cardiovascular fitness.

Procedures

1. Ride a stationary bicycle ergometer for six minutes at a rate of fifty pedal cycles per minute (one push with each foot per cycle).
2. Your instructor will set the work load of the bicycle depending on an estimation of your current exercise regularity. (Usually 300 to 900 KPM for women and 450 to 1,200 for men).
3. During the sixth minute of the ride your heart rate will be determined (the carotid pulse or the stethoscope will be used). For the test to be valid your heart rate must be in the range between 125 and 170 beats per minute.
4. Use the nomogram on page 157 to determine your predicted oxygen uptake score. Connect the point that represents your heart rate with the point on the right-hand scale that represents the work load you used in riding the bicycle (use the ♂ scale for men and the ♀ scale for women). Read your score at the point where a straight line connecting the two points crosses the Max VO₂ line. For example, the sample score for the woman represented by the dotted line is 2.55 or nearly 2.6. She had a heart rate of 150 and worked at a load of 600 KPM.

5. Check Chart 7.1 (page 158) to determine your cardiovascular fitness rating for the Max VO_2 (Maximum Oxygen Uptake) score obtained from the nomogram.
6. Determine your VO_2 per kilogram of body weight. Divide your body weight by 2.2. (This figure represents kilograms.) Divide this amount into your Max VO_2 score as determined from the nomogram. Locate your rating on Chart 7.1. This score will adjust your Max VO_2 for body weight and is a more accurate rating for people other than those of average weight.

Expected Results

Do you think you can easily ride a stationary bicycle against resistance for six minutes? Yes ☐ No ☐
Check your expected score on this cardiovascular fitness test.

Excellent	☐	Poor	☐
Very good	☐	Very Poor	☐
Marginal	☐		

Results

At what work load did you ride the bicycle? _____ KPM
What was your heart rate during the last minute of the ride? _____BPM
What was your score on the test? _____Liters of O_2
What was your score when corrected for body weight?_____ml/O_2/kg
What is your cardiovascular fitness rating on the bicycle test?
_____without weight adjustment
_____with weight adjustment

Conclusions and Implications

Did you score as well as you thought you would? Yes ☐ No ☐
Do you think this test indicates your true level of cardiovascular fitness? Yes ☐ No ☐
Are the ratings corrected for body weight different from the uncorrected rating? Yes ☐ No ☐
Explain.

What do the test results imply to you about your need for exercise?

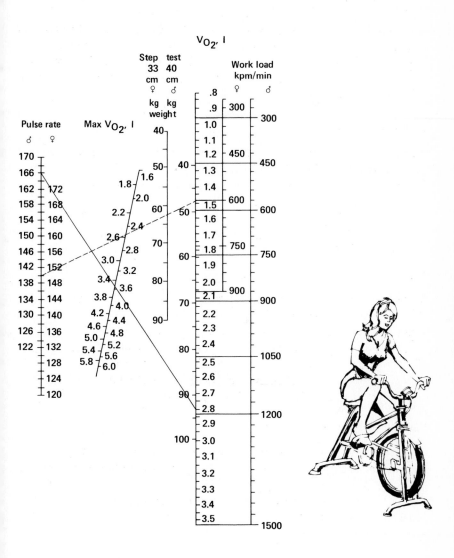

V_{O_2}, l

Step test
33 40
cm cm
♀   ♂

kg kg
weight

Work load
kpm/min
♀   ♂

Pulse rate   Max V_{O_2}, l

Chart 7.1 Bicycle Test Rating Scale*

Classification	Men		Women	
	O_2 in Liters	ML/O_2/KG	O_2 in Liters	ML/O_2/KG
Excellent	4.1+	54+	3.1+	47+
Very Good	3.3-4.0	46-53	2.6-3.0	42-46
Marginal	2.7-3.2	37-45	2.0-2.5	36-41
Poor	2.1-2.6	34-36	1.7-1.9	30-35
Very Poor	2.0 or below	33 or below	1.6 or below	29 or below

*You can continue to use this rating scale as you grow older.

Perform the four tests indicated below:

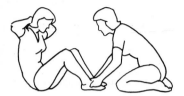

1. The bent knee sit-up. Lie on your back with the hands behind your head. Bend the knees at a 90° angle and have a partner hold your feet flat on the floor. Sit up, keeping the knees bent (see illustration). Lower the body to the starting position. You pass if you can do one!

2. Hanging leg-lift. Hang from a horizontal bar. Without swinging, *keeping the knees straight,* lift both legs until they touch the bar (see illustration). Lower the legs to the starting position. You pass if you can do one!

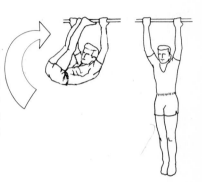

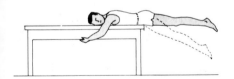

3. Lower trunk-lift. Lie prone on bench or table with legs hanging over the edge. Have a partner stabilize the upper back or grasp the edges of the table with the hands. Raise the legs parallel to the floor and lower them. *Do not raise past the horizontal or arch the back.* You pass if you can do one!

4. Upper trunk-lift. Lie on a table or bench with the upper half of the body hanging over the edge. Have a partner stabilize the feet while the trunk is raised parallel to the floor, then lower the trunk to the starting position. Place hands behind neck. *Do not raise past the horizontal or arch the back.* You pass if you do one!

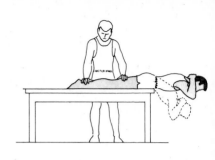

Record your results on page 159. To have *minimal* muscular strength you should pass *all* four tests.

Chart 9.1   Isometric Strength Rating Scale

Strength Rating Scale for Women

Classification	Left Grip	Right Grip	Back Strength	Leg Strength	Total Strength	Strength per/lb/wt
Excellent	82	90	245	300	714	5.50
Very Good	76-81	83-89	215-244	250-299	621-713	4.80-5.49
Marginal	48-75	56-82	115-214	145-249	361-620	2.90-4.79
Poor	40-47	49-55	86-114	86-114	258-360	2.10-2.89
Very Poor	below 39	below 48	below 85	below 85	below 257	below 200

Strength Rating Scale for Men

Classification	Left Grip	Right Grip	Back Strength	Leg Strength	Total Strength	Strength per/lb/wt
Excellent	150	155	460	530	1292	7.50
Very Good	124-149	136-154	390-459	470-529	1117-1291	7.10-7.49
Marginal	95-123	105-135	277-389	352-469	826-1116	5.21-7.09
Poor	86-94	91-104	201-276	301-351	676-825	4.81-5.20
Very Poor	below 85	below 90	below 200	below 300	below 675	below 4.80

*Because there is typically some loss of muscle tissue as you grow older, persons older than age 50 may wish to make an approximate 10 percent adjustment in the scores presented above.

Chart 10.1 Rating Scale for Flexed Arm Hang

Classification	Men		Women	
	Sitting tuck	Chins	Sitting tuck	Chins
Excellent	35	15	22	2
Very good	25	13	16	1
Adequate	12	7	8	—
Poor	8	4	5	—
Very poor	5		2	—

*Adjust scores downward by 10 percent after age fifty.

Chart 10.2 Rating Scale for Flexed Arm Hang
(for people who cannot do one chin)

Classification	Score in Seconds
Making progress toward chin up	25
Poor	12
Very Poor	8 or less

Evaluating Flexibility

Name _____ Section _____ Date _____

Flexibility is one of many important aspects of physical fitness. It is now clear that flexibility is of at least two types—dynamic and static—and is most likely specific to each body joint. For this reason, it is important that you perform exercises for each joint and each flexibility type if true flexibility is to be developed. Likewise, evaluation of flexibility should include tests for each joint and tests for both dynamic and static flexibility.

Purpose

The purpose of this laboratory session is to evaluate the flexibility of several body parts.

Procedures

1. Take the three tests as outlined on pages 173-174.
2. Record your scores in the "results" section.
3. Use Chart 11.1 on page 174 to determine your rating on each of the flexibility tests and record your rating in the "results" section.

Expected Results

How do you expect to score on the flexibility tests?

Excellent ☐   Poor ☐
Very good ☐   Very poor ☐
Marginal ☐

Results

	Test 1	Test 2	Test 3	
			Rt. up	Left up
What were your flexibility scores?	____	____	____	____
Record your flexibility rating.	____	____	____	____
(Use Chart 11.1 on page 174.)				

Conclusions and Implications

Did you score well on flexibility? Yes ☐ No ☐

Are you as flexible as you thought you were? Yes ☐ No ☐

On Test 3, did you score better with one arm up than with the other arm up? Yes ☐ No ☐

Do you need to perform flexibility exercises regularly? Yes ☐ No ☐

What flexibility exercises do you think you need to perform regularly?

Flexibility Tests

Since it is impractical to test the flexibility of all joints, perform these tests for the joints used most frequently in movement performance.

1. Upper Trunk and Shoulder Flexibility Test.*

   a. Stand with feet together and toes on the line on the floor with your side to the flexibility scale on the wall.

   b. Stand far enough from the wall so a closed fist can just touch the wall when the arm is horizontally extended.

   c. Extend the other arm to the side at shoulder height with palm down. Keeping the feet stationary, twist the trunk clockwise and reach as far as possible on the wall scale.

   d. The score is the point touched on the wall scale. Hold for at least two seconds.

   e. Repeat in the other direction.

2. Flexibility Test of Lower Back and Hamstrings

   a. Sit on the floor with the knees together and the feet flat against a bench turned on its side.

   b. With a partner holding the knees straight, reach forward with the arms fully extended.

   c. Measure the distance the fingertips reach on the yardstick fixed on the bench.

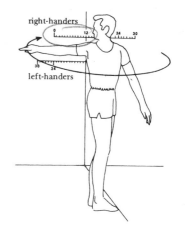

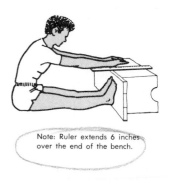

Note: Ruler extends 6 inches over the end of the bench.

*Edwin A. Fleischman, *The Structure and Measurement of Physical Fitness* (Englewood Cliffs, N. J.: Prentice-Hall, 1964), p. 162.

3. Shoulder Flexibility
   a. Stand with nose, chest, and abdomen against a projecting corner or a vertical pole.
   b. Raise the right arm, bend the elbow, and reach down across the back as far as possible.
   c. At the same time, extend the left arm down and behind the back, bend the elbow up the back and try to cross the fingers over those of the right hand.
   d. Measure the distance to the nearest half-inch. If fingers overlap score as a plus; if they fail to meet, score as a minus; use a zero if the fingertips just touch.
   e. Repeat with the arms crossed in the opposite direction (left arm up).

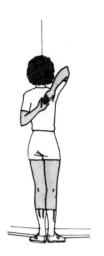

Chart 11.1 Flexibility Rating Scale*

Classification	Men				Women			
	Test 1	Test 2	Test 3		Test 1	Test 2	Test 3	
			R up	L up			R up	L up
Excellent	33	17	7	7	28	17	8	8
Very Good	28	13	6	5	25	14	7	6
Marginal	20	8	5	2	18	9	5	2
Poor	13	4	0	−2	13	4	0	−2
Very Poor	11	0	−2	−5	11	0	−2	−4

*Though many people become less flexible as they grow older, for optimal health, it is recommended that you attempt to maintain adequate levels of flexibility on the above chart throughout life.

Evaluating Body Fatness

Name_____Section_____Date_____

The critical factor in determining if a person is obese is whether the person has too much body fat rather than too much body weight. Unfortunately, the method most often used in determining obesity is the height-weight chart. In many cases this type of measure is inadequate. Thus, a height-weight chart might indicate that a highly muscular person is overweight. It is also possible for a "thin looking" person who possesses too much fat to be judged "normal" weight on a height-weight chart. The most practical method of determining body fatness is by the use of calipers for measuring skinfold thickness.

Purpose

The purpose of this laboratory session is to determine the percent of body fat possessed by each individual.

Procedures

1. Have your skinfold thicknesses measured as outlined on page 176.
2. Use nomogram 1 (women) or nomogram 2 (men) to determine your percent of body fat from your skinfold thickness scores. For women, locate your two skinfold scores on the appropriate scales of the nomogram. Read your percent of fat on the center scale. For men, follow the procedure located in the center of the nomogram.
3. Rate your "fatness" using Chart 12.1 on page 177. Record your percent of body fat and your body fat rating in the "results" section.

Results

What are your skinfold measurements?

Women			Men		
Iliac Crest	_____ mm		Abdomen	_____	mm
Triceps	_____ mm		Chest	_____	mm
			Triceps	_____	mm

What is your percent of body fat? _____ (Use Nomogram 1 or 2)

What is your fatness rating?

Very lean	☐	Fat	☐
Lean	☐	Obese	☐
Marginal	☐		

Conclusions and Implications

Does your percent body fat rating show you to be too fat? Yes ☐ No ☐
How do you account for your current body composition, and what do
   your results imply for you in the future?

Skinfold Tests

Take the following measures for women using a skinfold caliper. (See diagram.)

A. Triceps.

B. Illiac crest.

Take the following measures for men using a skinfold caliper. (See diagram.)

A. To right of navel.

B. Chest, above and to the right of the right nipple.

C. Triceps.

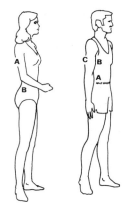

Note: All measurements are taken on the right side.

Chart 12.1   Fatness Rating Scale*

Classification	Men	Women
Very Lean	0-10	0-12
Lean	11-14	13-17
Marginal	15-17	18-22
Fat	18-19	23-27
Obese	20 plus	28 plus

*Though many people become fatter as they grow older, for optimal health, it is recommended that you attempt to maintain above marginal ratings of fatness throughout life.

Nomogram 1*

Nomogram for Conversion of Skinfold Thickness to Specific Gravity and Percent of Fat in Young Women

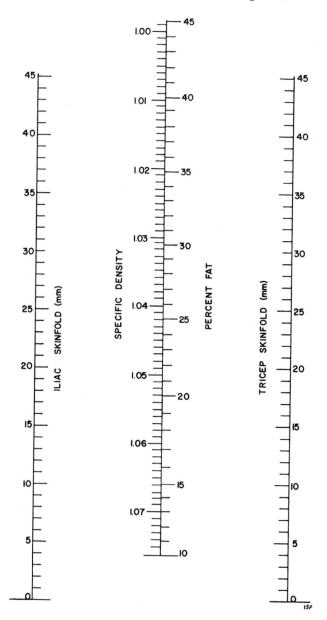

*Adapted from a nomogram by Irene Paul.

Nomogram 2*

Nomogram for Conversion of Skinfold Thickness
to Specific Gravity and Percent of Fat in Young Men

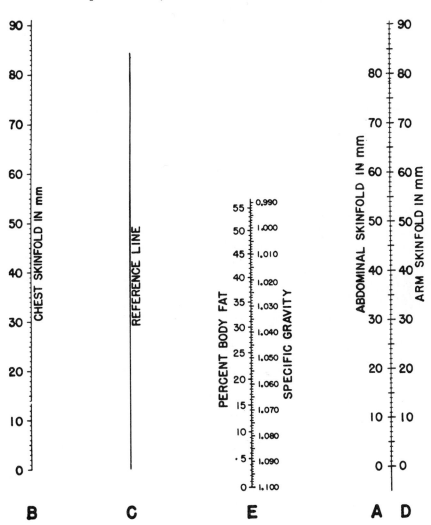

*Nomogram adapted from Consolazio, C. F., et al. *Physical Measurements of Metabolic Function in Man.* New York: McGraw-Hill, 1963 by permission.

Determining "Desirable" Body Weight

Name_____ Section_____ Date_____

Purpose

The purposes of this laboratory session are:

1. To determine "desirable" weight.
2. To compare two different methods for determining "desirable" body weight.

Procedures

1. Measure percent of body fat (see Lab 12), height, and weight. (Height without shoes and weight with indoor clothing).
2. Determine your frame size (small, medium, or large) using the following procedure. With a tape, measure the smallest girth of your wrist just above the styloid process (boney bump on wrist). Pull the tape snugly (but not tight enough to indent the skin) around the wrist as you measure. Look up your frame size on Chart 13.1.
3. Determine your "desirable" weight. Locate your height in inches on the left and your frame size across the top. Find the "desirable" weight for your height and frame size. Men use Chart 13.2; women use Chart 13.3.
4. Determine your "desirable" weight using a different procedure. Locate your actual body weight on the left and your percent body fat (from Lab 12) across the top. Find the "desirable" weight for your weight and body fat percent. Men use Chart 13.4; women use Chart 13.5.

Results

Record your scores below:

Percent body fat_____ Weight (indoor clothes) _____ lbs.

Height (without shoes)_____ inches

 Frame size   small ☐   medium ☐   large ☐

"Desirable" weight (Chart 13.1 or 13.2) _____ lbs.

"Desirable" weight (Chart 13.3 or 13.4) _____ lbs.

Conclusions and Implications

Is your "desirable" weight as determined from the height-weight chart above what it should be? Yes ☐ No ☐

Is your "desirable" weight as determined from percent body fat above what it should be? Yes ☐ No ☐

Is there a discrepancy between the answers above? Yes ☐ No ☐

If yes, why?

Using both "desirable" weights, what do you feel is the body weight you should have for the rest of your life? Explain. _____ lbs.

Chart 13.1 Determining Frame Size Using Wrist Size in Inches

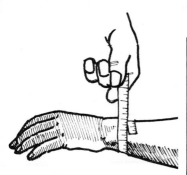

	Men	Women
Small frame	6½" or less	5½" or less
Medium frame	6¾"-7¼"	5¾"
Large frame	7½" or more	6" or more

Chart 13.2 Determination of "Desirable" Weight for Men*

Weight in Pounds According to Frame (in Indoor Clothing)			
Height (without shoes) Feet Inches	Small Frame	Medium Frame	Large Frame
5 1	112-120	118-129	126-141
5 2	115-123	121-133	129-144
5 3	118-126	124-136	132-148
5 4	121-129	127-139	135-152
5 5	124-133	130-143	138-156
5 6	128-137	134-147	142-161
5 7	132-141	138-152	147-166
5 8	136-145	142-156	151-170
5 9	140-150	146-160	155-174
5 10	144-154	150-165	159-179
5 11	148-158	154-170	164-184
6 0	152-162	158-175	168-189
6 1	156-167	162-180	173-194
6 2	160-171	167-185	178-199
6 3	164-175	172-190	182-204

Determining "Desirable" Body Weight

Chart 13.3 Determination of "Desirable" Weight for Women*

Weight in Pounds According to Frame (in Indoor Clothing)			
Height (without shoes) Feet Inches	Small Frame	Medium Frame	Large Frame
4 8	92- 98	96-107	104-119
4 9	94-101	98-110	106-122
4 10	96-104	101-113	109-125
4 11	99-107	104-116	112-128
5 0	102-110	107-119	115-131
5 1	105-113	110-122	118-134
5 2	108-116	113-126	121-138
5 3	111-119	116-130	125-142
5 4	114-123	120-135	129-146
5 5	118-127	124-139	133-150
5 6	122-131	128-143	137-154
5 7	126-135	132-147	141-158
5 8	130-140	136-161	145-163
5 9	134-144	140-155	149-168
5 10	138-148	144-159	153-173

*Tables adapted from those provided as a courtesy of the Metropolitan Life Insurance Co.

Determination of Desirable Body Weight for Men

Percent Fat

6	8	10	12	14	16	18	20	22	24	26	28	30	32	34	36	38	40
263	258	254	249	244	240	234	230	225	220	215	210	206	201	196	191	186	182
257	253	248	243	239	235	266	225	220	215	210	206	201	196	192	187	182	178
252	247	243	238	233	230	224	220	215	210	206	201	197	192	187	183	178	174
247	243	238	234	229	225	220	216	211	207	202	198	193	189	184	180	175	171
241	237	233	228	223	221	215	211	206	202	197	193	189	184	180	175	171	167
236	231	227	223	218	215	210	206	201	197	193	188	184	180	175	171	167	163
230	226	222	217	215	210	205	202	200	192	188	184	180	175	171	167	163	159
224	220	216	212	208	205	200	197	191	187	183	179	175	171	167	163	159	155
220	216	212	208	204	200	196	192	188	184	180	176	172	168	164	160	156	152
214	210	206	202	198	195	190	187	183	179	175	171	167	163	159	155	151	148
208	204	201	197	193	190	185	182	178	174	170	166	163	159	155	151	147	144
202	199	195	191	187	185	180	177	173	169	165	162	158	154	151	147	143	140
197	193	190	186	182	180	175	172	168	164	161	157	154	150	146	143	139	136
192	189	185	182	178	175	171	168	164	161	157	154	150	147	143	140	136	133
186	183	180	176	173	170	166	163	159	156	152	149	146	142	139	135	132	129
181	177	174	171	167	165	161	158	154	151	148	144	141	138	134	131	128	125
175	172	169	165	162	160	157	153	149	146	143	140	137	133	130	127	124	121
169	166	163	160	157	155	151	148	144	141	138	135	132	129	126	123	120	117
165	162	159	156	153	150	147	144	141	138	135	132	129	126	123	120	117	114
159	156	153	150	147	145	141	139	136	133	130	127	124	121	118	115	112	110
153	150	148	145	142	140	136	134	131	128	125	122	120	117	114	111	108	100
147	145	142	139	137	135	131	129	126	123	120	118	115	112	110	107	104	102
142	139	137	134	131	130	126	124	121	118	116	113	111	108	105	103	102	98
137	135	132	130	127	125	122	120	117	115	112	110	107	105	102	100	97	95
131	129	121	129	122	120	117	115	112	110	107	105	103	100	98	95	93	91

ong the side locate your actual body weight and across the top locate your estimated cent fat. The intersection of the two entries is your desirable weight (fat-free body ight plus 16 percent fat). Example: 175 pounds is the desirable weight for a man o weighs 195 pounds and currently has a body fat amount of 26 percent.

Chart 13.5 Determination of Desirable Body Weight for Women

Percent Fat

Actual Body Weight	6	8	10	12	14	16	18	20	22	24	26	28	30	32	34	36	38
200	228	224	220	216	212	208	204	200	196	192	188	184	180	176	172	168	164
195	222	218	214	210	206	202	198	195	191	187	183	179	175	171	167	163	159
190	216	212	209	205	201	197	193	190	186	182	178	174	171	167	163	159	155
185	210	207	203	199	196	192	188	185	181	177	173	170	166	162	159	155	151
180	205	201	198	194	190	187	183	180	176	172	169	165	162	158	154	151	147
175	199	196	192	189	185	182	178	175	171	168	164	161	157	154	150	147	143
170	193	180	177	173	170	166	163	170	166	163	159	156	153	149	146	142	139
165	188	184	181	178	174	171	168	165	161	158	155	151	148	145	141	138	135
160	182	179	176	172	169	166	163	160	156	153	150	147	144	140	137	134	131
155	176	173	170	167	164	161	158	155	151	148	145	142	139	136	133	130	127
150	171	168	165	162	159	156	153	150	147	144	141	138	135	132	129	126	123
145	165	162	159	156	153	150	147	145	142	139	136	133	130	127	124	121	118
140	159	156	154	151	148	145	142	140	137	134	131	128	126	123	130	117	114
135	153	151	148	145	143	140	137	135	132	129	126	124	121	118	116	113	110
130	148	145	143	140	137	135	132	130	127	124	122	119	117	114	111	109	106
125	142	140	137	135	132	130	127	125	122	120	117	115	112	110	107	105	102
120	136	134	132	129	127	124	122	120	117	115	112	110	108	105	103	100	98
115	131	128	126	124	121	119	117	115	112	110	108	105	103	101	98	96	94
110	125	123	121	118	116	114	112	110	107	105	103	101	99	96	94	92	90
105	119	117	115	113	111	109	107	105	102	100	98	96	94	92	90	88	86
100	114	112	110	108	106	104	102	100	98	96	94	92	90	88	86	84	82
95	108	106	104	102	100	98	96	95	93	91	89	87	85	83	81	79	77
90	102	100	99	97	95	93	91	90	88	86	84	82	81	79	77	75	73

Along the side locate your actual body weight and across the top locate your estimated percent fat. The intersection of the two entries is your desirable weight (fat-free body weight plus 20 percent fat). Example: 150 pounds is the desirable weight for a woman who weighs 160 pounds and currently has a body fat amount of 26 percent.

Exercise and Nutrition

Name_____Section_____Date_____

Purpose

The purposes of this laboratory session are:
1. To determine your caloric consumption during the morning.
2. To experience an exercise period that will expend as many calories as consumed at breakfast.
3. Relate caloric consumption (eating) to caloric expenditure (exercise).

Procedures

1. Determine what you ate for breakfast and record it on the blanks in the results section. (If you did not eat breakfast use a "typical" breakfast to complete this report).
2. Determine the calories consumed at breakfast using Chart 14.1, page 189, and record in the "results" section.
3. Walk, run, or swim until you have expended enough calories to equal the breakfast item with the fewest calories. Check that item off the list in the results section. Continue this procedure until all breakfast items are checked off or until the period is over.

Expected Results

Do you think you can expend your morning meal during the class period?
Yes ☐ No ☐

Results

List the foods you ate for breakfast below. Determine their calorie content from Chart 14.1 and record the calories next to the food. Check off each food as you exercise to expend enough calories (use Chart 14.1).

Breakfast Food	Calories	Check when expended by exercise
_____	_____	_____
_____	_____	_____
_____	_____	_____
_____	_____	_____
_____	_____	_____
_____	_____	_____

Conclusions and Implications

Did you think it would take more or less exercise to expend the calories in your breakfast? More ☐ Less ☐ Explain.

Do you feel that you exercise enough each day to expend the calories you eat? Yes ☐ No ☐

Do you feel that exercise alone is the method you could use to balance the calories you eat? Yes ☐ No ☐ Explain.

Chart 14.1 Minutes of Activity Necessary to Burn off Breakfast Foods

Breakfast Food	Calories	Number of Minutes of Activity Required to Burn Off Food			
		Walking	Swimming	Running	Sitting
Bacon (1 strip)	48	9	4	3	37
Beef (hamburger)	316	60	28	16	243
Bread and Butter	78	15	7	4	60
Candy Bar	300	58	27	15	230
Cantaloupe (raw)	60	12	5	3	46
Cereal (dry)	200	38	18	10	154
Coke (12 oz.)	137	26	12	7	105
Doughnut	151	29	13	8	116
Egg (fried)	125	24	11	6	96
Egg (boiled)	77	15	7	4	59
Egg (scrambled)	100	19	9	5	77
Grapefruit (fresh)	120	23	11	6	92
Grapefruit juice (1 cup)	95	18	8	5	73
Milk (1 glass)	166	32	15	9	128
Oatmeal (1 cup)	150	29	13	8	115
Orange	68	13	6	3	52
Orange juice (1 glass)	120	23	11	6	92
Pancake	59	11	5	3	45
Prune juice (1 cup)	170	33	15	9	131
Roll (sweet)	178	34	16	9	137

Exercise and Nutrition

Evaluating Balance Performance–
The Bass Test of Dynamic Balance

Name_____Section_____Date_____

The possession of motor skills is a desirable attribute. Although the possession of skills contributes less directly to physical health than do other aspects of physical fitness; the possession of skill can contribute to the development of a rich life. One who possesses skills can work more efficiently, enjoy leisure time through sports and games, and react positively to emergency situations. Some may choose to develop and maintain physical fitness through sports. One aspect of skill-related fitness is balance. For most people dynamic balance is the most important type of balance. Though the Bass Test is an old test, it is still considered a good test of dynamic balance.

Purpose

The purpose of this laboratory session is to evaluate your dynamic balance.

Procedures

1. Perform the Bass Test of Dynamic Balance as outlined on page 193.
2. Record your score in the results section.
3. Determine your balance rating from Chart 15.1 and record your rating in the "results" section.

Expected Results

How do you expect to score on this test of dynamic balance?

Excellent	☐	Poor	☐
Very good	☐	Very poor	☐
Marginal	☐		

Results

What is your balance score? _____
What is your balance rating? _____ (see Chart 15.1)

Conclusions and Implications

Did you perform as expected? Yes ☐ No ☐
Did you score well? Yes ☐ No ☐
Explain the reason for your test results.

What do the results imply to you for your daily life and recreational
  activities?

The Bass Test of Dynamic Balance*

Eleven circles (9½-inch) are drawn on the floor as pictured below.

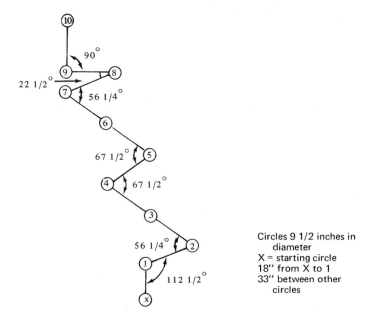

Circles 9 1/2 inches in
diameter
X = starting circle
18" from X to 1
33" between other
circles

The test is performed as follows:

1. Stand on the right foot in circle X. *Leap* forward to circle one, then circle two . . . through 10, alternating feet with each leap.
2. The feet must leave the floor on each leap and the heel may not touch. Only the ball of the foot may land on the floor.
3. Remain in each circle for five seconds before leaping to the next circle. (A count of five will be made for you, aloud).
4. Practice trials are allowed.
5. The score is fifty, plus the number of seconds taken to complete the test, minus the number of errors.
6. *All* errors are deducted at the rate of three points each. Errors include: touching the heel, moving the supporting foot, touching outside a circle, or touching any body part to the floor other than the supporting foot.
7. Scores should be plotted on the appropriate rating scales.

*From McCloy, C. H. *Tests and Measurements in Health and Physical Education.* New York: Appleton-Century-Crofts, 1954, p. 106.

Chart 15.1 Bass Test Rating Scale

Excellent	90-100
Very good	80- 89
Marginal	60- 79
Poor	30- 59
Very poor	0- 29

Evaluating Agility Performance– The Illinois Agility Run Test

Name_____Section_____Date_____

An important aspect of skill performance is agility; that is, the ability to change body positions quickly and accurately. The Illinois Agility Run is one method of testing agility.

Purpose

The purpose of this laboratory session is to evaluate your agility performance.

Procedures

1. Perform the Illinois Agility Run as outlined on page 197.
2. Record your running time in the "results" section.
3. Determine your agility rating from Chart 16.1, page 198, and record it in the "results" section.

Expected Results

How do you expect to score on this test of agility?

Excellent	☐	Poor	☐
Very good	☐	Very poor	☐
Marginal	☐		

Results

What is your agility run time? _____ seconds
What is your agility rating? _____ (see Chart 16.1)

Conclusions and Implications

Did you perform as expected? Yes ☐ No ☐
Did you score well? Yes ☐ No ☐
Explain the reason for your test results.

What do the results imply to you for your daily life and recreational activities?

The Illinois Agility Run*

An agility course using four chairs and a thirty-foot running area will be set up as depicted in the illustration.

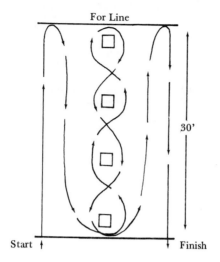

The test is performed as follows:

1. Lie prone with the hands by the shoulders and with the head at the starting line. On the signal to begin, the performer will run the course as fast as possible.
2. The performer's score is the time required to complete the course.

*Adams, et al. *Foundations of Physical Activity* (Champaign, Ill.: Stipes and Co., 1965), p. 111.

Chart 16.1 Agility Rating Scale

Classification	Men	Women
Excellent	15.8 or faster	17.4 or faster
Very good	16.7 - 15.9	18.6 - 17.5
Marginal	18.6 - 16.8	22.3 - 18.7
Poor	18.8 - 18.7	23.4 - 22.4
Very poor	18.0 or slower	23.5 or slower

Evaluating Explosive Power– The Standing Long Jump

Name_____Section_____Date_____

Explosive power is an aspect of fitness that is defined as strength times speed; in other words, strength feats that are performed explosively or quickly. An example of explosive power is the standing long jump.

Purpose

The purpose of this laboratory session is to evaluate your explosive power.

Procedures

1. Perform the Standing Long Jump Test as outlined on page 200.
2. Record your distance score in the "results" section.
3. Determine your explosive power rating from Chart 17.1 and record it in the "results" section.

Expected Results

How do you expect to score on this test of explosive power?

Excellent	☐	Poor	☐
Very good	☐	Very poor	☐
Marginal	☐		

Results

Record your standing long jump score. _____ inches
What is your explosive power rating? _____ (see Chart 17.1)

Conclusions and Implications

Did you perform as expected? Yes ☐ No ☐
Did you score well? Yes ☐ No ☐
Explain the reason for your test results.

What do the results imply for your daily life and recreational activities?

The Standing Long Jump Test

The test is performed as follows:

1. Stand with both feet behind a starting line.
2. Jump forward with both feet as far as possible.
3. Measure the jump distance to the point where the body touched nearest the take off line.
4. Your score is the best of three jumps.

Chart 17.1   Power Rating Scale

Classification	Men	Women
Excellent	8'6" +	6'8" +
Very good	7'9"-8'5"	5'10"-6'7"
Marginal	6'4"-7'8"	4'8"-5'9"
Poor	5'10"-6'3"	4'2"-4'7"
Very poor	Below 5'9"	Below 4'1"

Evaluating Coordination— The Stick Test of Coordination

Name_____Section_____Date_____

Coordination is the ability to use the senses together with the body parts. The stick test is one method of evaluating hand-eye coordination.

Purpose

The purpose of this laboratory session is to evaluate your coordination.

Procedures

1. Perform the Stick Test of Coordination as outlined on page 203.
2. Record your score in the "results" section.
3. Determine your coordination rating from Chart 18.1, page 204, and record it in the "results" section.

Expected Results

How do you expect to score on this test of coordination?

Excellent	☐	Poor	☐
Very good	☐	Very poor	☐
Marginal	☐		

Results

Record your coordination score. _____
What is your coordination rating? _____ (see Chart 18.1)

Conclusions and Implications

Did you perform as well as expected? Yes ☐ No ☐
Did you score well? Yes ☐ No ☐
Explain the reason for your test results.

What do the results imply to you for your daily life and recreational
   activities?

Do you think you could improve your coordination with practice?
   Yes ☐ No ☐

How much improvement would you expect? Discuss.

The Stick Test of Coordination

The Stick Test of Coordination requires you to juggle with three wooden wands. The wands are used to perform a one half flip and a full flip.

1. One Half Flip—Hold two twenty-four inch (one-half inch in diameter) dowel rods, one in each hand. Support a third twenty-four inch rod across the other two. Toss the supported rod in the air so that it makes a half turn. Catch the thrown rod with the two held rods.

2. Full Flip—Perform the above task letting the supported rod turn a full flip.

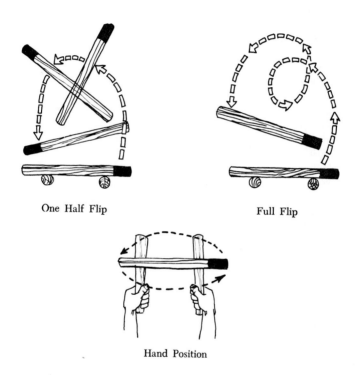

One Half Flip   Full Flip

Hand Position

The test is performed as follows:

1. Practice a half flip and the full flip several times before taking the test.
2. When you are ready, attempt a half flip five times. Score one point for each successful attempt.
3. When you are ready, attempt the full flip five times. Score two points for each successful attempt.

Chart 18.1 Coordination Rating Scale

Classification	Men	Women
Excellent	14-15	13-15
Very good	11-13	10-12
Marginal	5-10	4- 9
Poor	3- 4	2- 3
Very poor	0- 2	0- 1

Body Mechanics

19

Name_____Section_____Date_____

There are some general principles of good body mechanics that should be observed when giving and receiving force, but within that framework, there are a variety of correct methods. There is no one best method that applies in every situation. One must consider all of the factors involved in a specific problem and choose the procedure that best accomplishes the job. Remember the criteria: efficiency, effectiveness, and safety.

Purpose

The purposes of this laboratory session are:
1. To provide an opportunity to practice pushing, pulling, lifting, carrying, and the principles of stability.
2. To provide an opportunity to experiment with a number of methods in order to evaluate the effects.
3. To provide an opportunity for experimenting with a number of objects varying in weight, size, shape, and friction in order to determine the effect of these factors on body mechanics.

Procedures

A. Choose a partner of similar size. Stand facing, palms of hands together, legs in a front stride position, knees bent in a half-crouch.
   1. Try to push partner backward; keep the back straight, use the leg muscles, and lean forward. Try it with arms straight and then with arms bent. The opponent should attempt to remain stable and resist being moved.
   2. Same as above except try to pull partner forward as you move backward.
   3. Same as above, except try pushing and pulling while facing sideward; push while facing backward; pull while facing forward.
B. Using a blanket, beach towel, mat, or gym scooter, pull partner across the floor while he/she sits on the "chariot."
   1. Using good body mechanics, face partner and walk backwards.
   2. Face away from the partner and walk forward.
   3. Face sideward and walk sideward.

4. Grasp the blanket (rope or handle) close to the partner, making a short handle, while pulling.
5. Lengthen the handle and note the difference in pulling.

C. Practice lifting, carrying, and lowering a variety of objects that the instructor has placed around the room.

D. One partner assumes a stable position; the other partner should place his/her hands on his/her shoulders and try to push or pull him/her off balance without revealing the intended direction.

Results

Which seems best?

1. Pushing ☐   Pulling ☐
2. Bent arm pushing ☐   Straight arm pushing ☐
3. Backward ☐   Forward ☐   Sideward ☐

Which way seemed best for pulling the "chariot"?

1. Forward ☐   Backward ☐   Sideward ☐
2. Long handle ☐   Short handle ☐

Which factors were important in pushing and pulling?

	Most Important	Next in Importance	Least Important
Size	☐	☐	☐
Shape	☐	☐	☐
Weight	☐	☐	☐
Location in Space	☐	☐	☐

What did you do to your base to improve stability?
Lengthen ☐ Widen ☐ Narrow ☐ Diagonal ☐

What did you do to the center of gravity to improve stability?
Raise ☐ Lower ☐ Shift toward force ☐ Shift away from force ☐
Keep centered ☐

Conclusions and Implications

Explain the implications of the above questions to a daily life activity or to a sport. Examples: blocking in football, pushing a stalled car, or carrying a forty-pound suitcase in an airport.

Body Mechanics in Sports

Name_____ Section_____ Date_____

Just as in daily life, there are certain principles of movement that can be used in sports to make you more efficient. These principles are considered to be the Principles of Body Mechanics.

Purpose

The purposes of this laboratory session are:

1. To show that sports performance can be improved by following the Principles of Body Mechanics.

2. To demonstrate with one sports skill (jumping) how proper body mechanics can improve performance.

3. To identify some of the principles of body mechanics in actual sports situations.

Procedures

With a partner, practice jumping five different ways as described below. Use the best of three tries as your score for each different way of jumping. Record your scores for each jump in the results section.

Perform the five jumps (standing long jump) as follows:

1. With both feet behind a starting line, jump forward with both feet as far as possible.
   a. Jump 1—Do the jump with the arms held crossed against the chest.
   b. Jump 2—Do the jump with the arms held tightly against your sides.
   c. Jump 3—Throw the arms vigorously in the air as you jump.
   d. Jump 4—Take one short hop from behind the line before jumping; swing the arms up.
   e. Jump 5—Take one short hop before jumping but keep the arms at your sides.

2. Measure the jump distance to the point where the body touched nearest the take-off line.

Expected Results

Before you do the five jumps read how each is to be performed.
On which jump do you expect to perform best?
    1 ☐ 2 ☐ 3 ☐ 4 ☐ 5 ☐
On which jump do you expect to perform worst?
    1 ☐ 2 ☐ 3 ☐ 4 ☐ 5 ☐

Results

What was your score on each of the five jumps?

Jump 1 _____ inches
Jump 2 _____ inches
Jump 3 _____ inches
Jump 4 _____ inches
Jump 5 _____ inches

Conclusions and Implications

Did you perform best on the jump expected? Yes ☐ No ☐
Were you able to jump equally far on every attempt? Yes ☐ No ☐
  If not, why not?

On which attempt did you jump the farthest? 1 ☐ 2 ☐ 3 ☐ 4 ☐ 5 ☐
  Why?

Explain the reasons why you did better or poorer on different attempts,
  and tell what mechanical principles were involved.

Posture

Name _____ Section _____ Date _____

Purposes

The purposes of this laboratory session are as follows:
1. To learn to recognize postural deviations and thus become more posture conscious.
2. To determine one's own faults in order that a preventive and corrective program might be instituted.

Procedures

1. Wear as little clothing as possible (bathing suits are recommended) and remove shoes and socks.
2. Work in groups of two or three, with one person acting as the "subject" while partners serve as "examiners"; alternate roles.
3. Use the Posture Evaluation Chart 21.1 (page 211) to determine your posture score.
4. Rate your posture score on the rating Chart 21.2 (page 211).

Expected Results

What do you expect your posture rating to be?

Excellent ☐   Poor ☐
Very good ☐   Very poor ☐
Marginal ☐

Results

Record your posture score. _____
Record your posture rating. _____

Conclusions

Were you aware of the deviations that were found? Yes ☐ No ☐
List the deviations that were moderate or severe.

Implications

What will you do about your postural faults? List specific exercises (or habits) you need to practice to correct each deviation listed in the "conclusion" above. If you were checked as having some of the symptoms of scoliosis, see your instructor for a more thorough examination and possible referral to a physician.

Evaluating Posture

There is probably no one best posture for all individuals, but there are some basic and common posture problems that can be relatively easily identified.

Procedures

1. Stand by a vertically hung plumb line.
2. Using the Posture Evaluation Chart check the deviations found by indicating their severity as follows: 0—none; 1—slight; 2—moderate; 3—severe.
3. Total the score and determine your posture rating on the chart provided for the laboratory.

Chart 21.1   Posture

Side View	Points	Back View	Points
Head Forward	_____	Tilted Head	_____
Sunken Chest	_____	Protruding Scapulae	_____
Round Shoulders	_____	Symptoms of Scoliosis:	
Kyphosis	_____	Shoulders Uneven	_____
Lordosis	_____	Hips Uneven	_____
Abdominal Ptosis	_____	Lateral Curvature of Spine (Adams Position)	_____
Hyperextended Knees	_____		
Body Lean	_____	One Side of Back is High (Adams Position)	_____

Total Score _____

Chart 21.2   Posture Rating Scale

Classification	Total Score
Excellent	0-2
Very Good	3-4
Marginal	5-7
Poor	8-11
Very Poor	12 or more

During this Lab, you will take three simple tests.

Tests for Muscular Imbalance

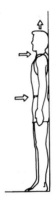

1. **Back-Wall Test.** Stand with the back against a wall, with head, heels, shoulders, and calves of legs touching the wall. Try to flatten the neck and hollow of your back by pressing your buttocks down against the wall. Your partner should just be able to place a hand in the space between the wall and the small of your back. If this space is greater than the thickness of his hand, you probably have lordosis with shortened lumbar and hip flexor muscles.

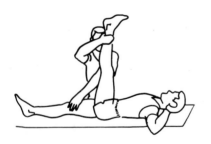

2. **Supine Leg Lift.** Lie on your back with hands behind your neck. The partner on your right should stabilize your right leg by placing his/her left hand on the knee. With the right hand, your partner should grasp the left ankle and raise the left leg as near to a right angle as possible. In this position, the lower back should be in contact with the floor. The right leg should remain straight and on the floor throughout the test. If the left leg bends at the knee, short hamstring muscles are indicated. If the back arches and/or the right leg does not remain flat on the floor, short lumbar muscles or hip flexor muscles (or both) are indicated. Repeat the test on the opposite side.

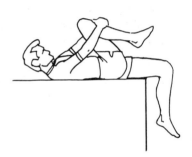

3. **Knee to chest.** Lie on your back on a table or bench with the right leg extended beyond the edge of the table (approximately one-third of thigh off of table). Bring left knee to chest and pull it down tightly with hands. The lower back should remain flat against the table. Right thigh should remain on table. If the right thigh lifts off the table while the left knee is hugged to chest, a tight hip flexor (iliopsoas) on that side is indicated. Repeat on opposite side.

Care of the Back

Name_____ Section_____ Date_____

Purpose

The purpose of this laboratory session is to determine if you have some muscle imbalance and to learn exercises suitable for preventing backaches and correcting lordosis.

Procedures

1. Secure a partner and administer the three muscle tests to each other. (For details see page 212.) Record results of tests in the "results" section of this report.

2. Under the direction and supervision of the instructor, perform the exercises described on pages 266-268. Two or three repetitions of each will be adequate for the purposes of this laboratory.

Expected Results

Do you have any back problems? Yes ☐ No ☐

Do you expect to have any difficulty with the tests of back weakness? Yes ☐ No ☐

Results and Conclusions

1. On Test number 1, was there evidence that you have shortened lumbar and/or hip flexor muscles? Yes ☐ No ☐

2. (a) On Test number 2, was there evidence that you have short hamstrings?
   Yes ☐ No ☐   Right ☐ Left ☐

   (b) Was there evidence of short lumbar and/or hip flexor muscles?
   Yes ☐ No ☐

3. On Test number 3, was there evidence that you have short hip flexors?
   Yes ☐ No ☐   Right ☐ Left ☐

4. Did you have difficulty performing any of the exercises? Yes ☐ No ☐
   If so, which ones?

How do you account for this difficulty?

Implications

If your answers to the questions are positive, what does this suggest to
   you in terms of your susceptibility to backache?
What specific exercises might help solve these problems?

Stress

Name _____ Section _____ Date _____

The purpose of this laboratory session is to determine the amount of stress resulting from the application of various physical and emotional stressors.

One method of measuring stress is heart rate. Although increase in heart rate can represent the desirable effects of physical overload on the heart, it can also reflect wear and tear on the heart as a result of constant demands that are not part of a plan of progressive overload. These constant demands produce stress that prevents desirable and necessary heart rest. Stress is also reflected in the rate of wear and tear on other body systems.

Purposes

The purposes of this laboratory session are as follows:

1. To identify the relative stress caused by different physical and emotional stressors.
2. To determine the amount of time required to recover from the various stressors.

Procedures

Determine your resting heart rate. Next you will be exposed to five different stressors. After each stressor is applied count your heart rate for thirty seconds. Allow three minutes to lower the heart rate after each stressor. Record your heart rates for each stressor in the results section. Exchange data with another student so that records can be compared.

Expected Results*

Which do you think will cause the greatest increase in heart rate?
　　　　Emotional Stressors ☐　　　　Physical Stressors ☐
Who do you think will have the biggest heart rate change under stress?
　　　　　　You ☐　　　　Your partner ☐

*NOTE: Typically women will have slightly higher resting heart rates than men.

Results

Record stressors and thirty second heart rates on the chart below.

Stressor	Heart Rate	
	Self	Partner
1.		
2.		
3.		
4.		
5.		

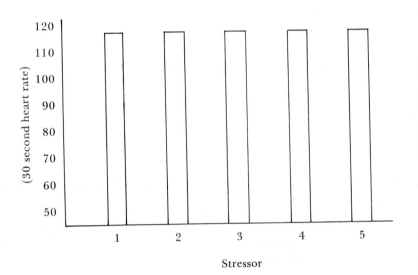

Darken the bar for each of the five stressors to indicate heart rate after each of the stressors are applied.

Conclusions and Implications

Did your partner react to the stress in the same way as you did?
Yes ☐ No ☐ Explain.

Does previous experience affect the way you respond to stress?
Yes ☐ No ☐ Explain.

Explain the fact that some people do not experience much stress from physical exercise.

Tension, Relaxation, and Tension Relieving Exercise

Name _____ Section _____ Date _____

Purpose

The purpose of this laboratory session is to learn to recognize signs of excess tension in oneself and in others by observation of symptomatic mannerisms and by manually testing ability to relax. If time permits, perform the relaxation exercises on page 269 before executing the lab.

Procedures

1. Choose a partner; designate one partner as the subject and the other as the tester. Alternate roles.
2. The subject should lie supine in a comfortable position and try to consciously relax as described in Concept 10. An individual may do this alone, or the instructor may wish to direct the entire group in this procedure.
3. The tester should kneel beside the subject's right hand and remain very still and quiet, while the subject is concentrating.
4. After five minutes have elapsed, the tester should observe the subject for signs of tension according to the procedures outlined on page 220.
5. Record your relaxation rating in the results section of this report. (Use Chart 24.1 to determine your rating).

Expected Results

Are you a tense person? Yes ☐ No ☐
What will your tension-relaxation rating be?

Relaxed	☐	Moderately tense	☐
Mildly tense	☐	Markedly tense	☐

Results

Record your tension score. _____
Rate yourself in relaxation. (Use the Rating Scale on page 222.) _____

Conclusions and Implications

Were you aware of your own tensions? Yes ☐ No ☐

Was it more difficult to relax than you expected? Yes ☐ No ☐

Did your awareness of your partner make it more difficult to concentrate? Yes ☐ No ☐

Can you concentrate on your breathing without altering its rhythm? Yes ☐ No ☐

Could you learn to consciously release muscular tension with additional practice? Yes ☐ No ☐

Could you learn to release tension with your eyes open while sitting or standing? Yes ☐ No ☐

What implications does this concept have for you in terms of your daily life (e.g., sleeping, studying, taking exams, performing on stage, etc.).

Evaluating Muscular Tension

A trained person can diagnose neuromuscular hypertension by observation and by manual testing. There is insufficient time in this course to master either the technique of relaxing or the evaluation techniques, but it is possible to learn the procedures for both.

Procedures

1. Following the procedures outlined on page 219, look for visual signs of tension outlined in section A on the chart. Place a check mark in the appropriate column.

2. Quietly and gently, the tester should grasp the subject's right wrist with his fingers, and slowly raise it about three inches from the floor, letting it hinge at the elbow; then let the hand drop. Observe signs of tension in section B of the chart. Record results.

3. After all visual and manual symptoms have been recorded on the chart, determine the total number of symptoms checked "yes."
4. Find your total score on the rating chart to determine your rating (see Chart 24.1).

Signs of Tension

	No	Yes
A. Visual Symptoms 1. Frowning		✓
2. Twitching		✓
3. Eyelids flutter		
4. Breathing a. shallow		
b. rapid		
c. irregular		✓
5. Mouth tight		✓
6. Swallowing		✓
B. Manual Symptoms 1. Assistance (subject helps lift arm)		
2. Resistance (subject resists movement)		
3. Posturing (subject holds arm in raised position)		
4. Perseveration (subject continues upward movement)		

Total number of "yes" checks. _____

Chart 24.1 Tension-Relaxation Rating Scale

Classification	Total Score
Excellent (relaxed)	0
Very Good (mild tension)	1 - 3
Marginal (moderate tension)	4 - 6
Poor (tense)	7 - 9
Very Poor (marked tension)	10 - 12

A Cardiovascular Fitness Program–Aerobics

Name_____ Section_____ Date_____

Some of the cardiovascular health benefits that are purported to result from regular progressive exercise include the development of a stronger heart muscle, healthier arteries, lower resting heart rate, better oxygen supply to working muscles (including the heart) and improved coronary collateral circulation. One program that claims all of these benefits is the Aerobics program developed by Dr. Kenneth Cooper.

Purpose

The purposes of this laboratory session are:

1. To give you an opportunity to experience a part of an exercise program designed to develop cardiovascular fitness.
2. To familiarize you with an exercise program that can be continued as part of your normal life's pattern.

Procedures

1. Read about the Aerobics Program on pages 107-108.
2. Select one aerobics activity and perform it earning as many aerobics points as you can during the laboratory period.

Expected Results

Will you be able to earn three to six points without undue fatigue?
Yes ☐ No ☐
Is thirty minutes enough time to spend in earning the desired number of points? Yes ☐ No ☐

Results

What activity did you choose to perform? _____
How many points did you earn? _____
How many days a week would you have to do the same exercise to earn thirty points a week? _____

Conclusions and Implications

Did you do as well as expected? Yes ☐ No ☐
Was the exercise within your level of capacity? Yes ☐ No ☐ Explain.

Would the Aerobics program be a good fitness program for YOU?
Yes ☐ No ☐
Do you think you will continue this type of program? Yes ☐ No ☐ Why?

The Adult Fitness Program

Name _____ Section _____ Date _____

The President's Council on Physical Fitness and Sport has developed a complete progressive exercise program. A special book titled *Adult Physical Fitness* outlines several exercise programs that range from very simple to quite difficult. The manual suggests that an individual do a self-test and then begin with the program that best meets his or her individual needs.

Purpose

The purposes of this laboratory session are:

1. To give you an opportunity to experience a part of an exercise program designed to develop total physical fitness.
2. To acquaint you with an exercise program that can be continued as part of your normal life's pattern.

Procedures

1. Read about the Adult Physical Fitness Program on page 108.
2. Perform the sample program described on pages 272-274.

Results

Did you complete the program of exercises in thirty minutes? Yes ☐ No ☐
If not, how much more time did you need? _____ minutes

Conclusions and Implications

Was the program too easy? Yes ☐ No ☐
Was it too difficult? Yes ☐ No ☐ Explain.

Will the *Adult Fitness Program* be a good one for you? Yes ☐ No ☐
Do you think *you* would continue this type of program? Yes ☐ No ☐
  Why?

The XBX and 5BX Physical Fitness Programs

Name _____ Section _____ Date _____

The Royal Canadian Air Force developed the XBX plan of exercise for women and the 5BX for men to help air force personnel become and stay physically fit. Since the time of the program's development, many lay people have selected the XBX and 5BX programs as their regular exercise program.

Purpose

The purposes of this laboratory session are:

1. To give you an opportunity to experience a part of an exercise program designed to develop total physical fitness.
2. To familiarize you with an exercise program that can be continued as part of your normal life's pattern.

Procedures

1. Read about the XBX and 5BX programs on page 108.
2. Perform the sample program described on pages 274-278.

Results

How long did it take you to complete the program of exercises? _____ minutes

Was the program too easy? Yes ☐ No ☐
Too difficult? Yes ☐ No ☐ Explain.

Conclusions and Implications

Will the Royal Canadian Air Force XBX or 5BX be a good program for you? Yes ☐ No ☐

Would you like to continue this type program? Yes ☐ No ☐ Why or why not?

A Progressive Rhythmical Endurance Exercise Program

Name_____ Section_____ Date_____

When an individual attempts to find a personal exercise program that best meets his/her own fitness needs the individual should consider the following criteria (1) will the program help improve or maintain *all* of the health-related aspects of fitness, and (2) is the program interesting enough to stimulate continued participation. One program that meets the above criteria is a progressive rhythmical endurance circle exercise program. The following program has been used quite successfully with adult groups. In fact, research shows that persons participating in these exercises for six to ten weeks show significant improvements in *all* aspects of health-related fitness. Those who have used these circle exercises acknowledged that persons who begin this type of program are likely to continue, especially if several people organize to perform the exercise as a group.

Purpose

The purposes of this laboratory session are:

1. To give you an opportunity to experience an exercise program designed to develop the health-related aspects of physical fitness with emphasis on cardiovascular fitness.
2. To acquaint you with an exercise program that can be continued as part of your normal life's pattern.

Procedures

1. Read about the program on pages 108-109.
2. Perform the program. You may choose to exercise ten, fifteen, or twenty minutes depending on your level of fitness (pages 278-280).

Results

Were you able to complete the entire exercise program? Yes ☐ No ☐

Conclusions and Implications

Did you exercise as long as you expected? Yes ☐ No ☐

What is your feeling concerning the advantages and disadvantages of this type of an exercise program?

Do you think circle exercises would be a good fitness program for you? Yes ☐ No ☐ Why or why not?

Do you think you will continue this type program later in life? Yes ☐ No ☐ Why or why not?

Circuit Training

Name_____Section_____Date_____

Circuit Training is a method of training that involves moving from place to place to perform different exercises designed to develop different aspects of physical fitness. Circuit training was popularized by two Englishmen in the early 1960s, though this method of training has been used for many years.

Purpose

The purposes of this laboratory session are:

1. To give you an opportunity to experience a circuit training program designed to increase several components of physical fitness.
2. To acquaint you with a training program that can be continued throughout your life.

Procedures

1. Read about the program on page 109.
2. Perform the program as described on pages 280-282.

Results

Were you able to complete the program for thirty minutes? Yes ☐ No ☐
If not, how long would it take?_____ minutes.

Conclusions and Implications

Was the circuit training program a good one for you? Yes ☐ No ☐
If not, do you prefer some stations to others in the circuit? Yes ☐ No ☐
Which ones?

Do you think you would continue this type of program for use later in life? Yes ☐ No ☐ Why?

Speed Play or Fartlek

Name_____ Section_____ Date_____

This type of program, originally developed in Sweden, is a combination of fast running, slow running, walking, and a limited number of fast calisthenics. Though designed originally as a training technique for athletes it has been adapted as a program for people just interested in improving their fitness.

Purpose

The purposes of this laboratory session are:

1. To give you an opportunity to experience an exercise program designed to develop cardiovascular fitness and to a lesser extent other aspects of health-related physical fitness.
2. To acquaint you with an exercise program that can be continued as part of your normal life's pattern.

Procedures

1. Read about the "Speed Play" program on page 109.
2. Perform the program. You may choose to walk or jog instead of performing all of the exercises if the program is too vigorous for your current level of fitness (pages 282-283).

Results

Were you able to complete the entire "Speed Play" program? Yes ☐ No ☐

Interval Training

Name _____ Section _____ Date _____

Interval Training is the name used to describe a method of "anaerobic" or Intermittent Exercise Training. Originally developed as a method of conditioning for athletes it is now used by many individuals as part of their regular program for physical fitness development. Interval Training involves running relatively short distances at a relatively high intensity followed by low intensity running or resting.

Purpose

The purposes of this laboratory session are:

1. To give you an opportunity to experience interval training or an anaerobic exercise program for developing cardiovascular fitness.
2. To familiarize you with an interval training program that can be continued for a lifetime.

Procedures

1. Read about Interval Training on page 110.
2. Perform the sample Interval Training Program (pages 283-284).

Results

Were you able to complete the entire Interval Training Program?
Yes ☐ No ☐ If not, how long were you able to continue? _____

Conclusions and Implications

Was the Interval Training Program a good one for you? Yes ☐ No ☐
If not, do you prefer the aerobics? Yes ☐ No ☐
Anaerobics? Yes ☐ No ☐

Do you think you would continue this type of program? Yes ☐ No ☐
Why?

What type of an Interval Training Program would be best for you? Describe.

Jogging

Name_____Section_____Date_____

Jogging is a form of aerobic exercise that has become extremely popular as a method of developing cardiovascular fitness. It has a major advantage in that it does not require a great deal of skill and for this reason almost any individual can enjoy the benefits of this form of exercise.

Purpose

The purposes of this laboratory session are:

1. To give you an opportunity to experience one type of jogging program that can be used to develop and maintain cardiovascular fitness.
2. To acquaint you with the basic techniques of jogging.

Procedures

1. Work with a partner and rate each other on the jogging techniques. Make a note on Chart 32.1 if you have any problems in your technique.
2. Using proper jogging technique, jog for fifteen minutes at your own individual cardiovascular threshold of training. (Determine your threshold of training from Chart 4.1, page 147.)

Results

What is your cardiovascular threshold of training? _____ bpm
What was your heart rate after your fifteen minute jog? _____ bpm
During your fifteen minute jog did you reach your threshold of training?
   Yes ☐ No ☐
With the help of a partner, note any problems in technique in the following chart. (Read the jogging information on page 284 before rating your partners jogging technique.

Chart 32.1   Jogging Technique

Source of Problem	Severity of Problem	
	none	needs work
Foot Placement		
Length of Stride		
Arm Movement		
Body Position		

Do you feel that you can solve any jogging problems you have? Yes ☐
No ☐ No problems ☐

Conclusions and Implications

Do you think that jogging is a good type of exercise for you? Yes ☐ No ☐
Explain.

Do you think that you will include jogging in your exercise program for use in later life? Yes ☐ No ☐ Explain.

Weight Training or Isotonic Exercise

Name_____ Section_____ Date_____

Weight training is a type of isotonic exercise that requires you to lift a weighted bar or dumbbell in order to overload specific muscles. Recent evidence indicates weight training is appropriate for both men and women.

Purpose

The purposes of this laboratory session are:

1. To give you an opportunity to experience a sample weight training program.
2. To acquaint you with a strength program that can be continued throughout your life.

Procedures

1. Read about weight training on page 110.
2. Perform the weight training exercises using the weights and repetitions listed below. (This is a sample program that would have to be modified to meet your individual needs as described on page 285. The *sample program* is *not* intended as a program for regular use.)

Sample Program

Weight Training *

Exercise	Sets	Repetitions	Beginning Wt. Men	Beginning Wt. Women
Shoulder Shrug	3	6	60 pounds	40 pounds
Military Press	3	6	50 pounds	40 pounds
Half Knee Squats	3	6	60 pounds	40 pounds
Curls	3	6	40 pounds	30 pounds
Forearm Extension Behind Neck	3	6	25 pounds	15 pounds
Toe Raises	3	6	60 pounds	40 pounds
Pull to Chin	3	6	30 pounds	20 pounds

*For exercise details see pages 286-289.

Results

How long did it take you to complete the program? _____ minutes
Was the program too long? Yes ☐ No ☐
Too easy? Yes ☐ No ☐
Too difficult? Yes ☐ No ☐ Explain.

Conclusions and Implications

Will the weight training be a good program for you? Yes ☐ No ☐
Would you like to continue this type program? Yes ☐ No ☐ Why or
  why not?

Isometric Exercise

Name_____Section_____Date_____

Isometric exercises were first popularized by German scientists and later used extensively by coaches for preparation for football. This type exercise has since been adapted for use in regular exercise programs. Isometrics involve static contractions of the muscles with no movement of the body parts.

Purpose

The purposes of this laboratory session are:

1. To give you an opportunity to experience a sample isometric exercise program.
2. To acquaint you with strength exercises that you may wish to include as a part of your exercise program for a lifetime.

Procedures

1. Read about isometric exercises on pages 34-35.
2. Perform the isometric exercises, repetitions and durations suggested below. (This is a sample program that needs to be modified to meet your individual needs as described on page 289. The sample program is *not* intended as a program for regular use.)

Sample Program

Isometric Exercises *

Exercise	Repetitions	Duration
Shoulder Pull	3	8 seconds
Chest Push	3	8 seconds
Curl	3	8 seconds
Wall Seat	3	8 seconds
Leg Extension	3	8 seconds

*For exercise details see pages 290-294.

Results

Was the program too hard? Yes ☐ No ☐
Too easy? Yes ☐ No ☐ Explain.

Conclusions and Implications

Will isometrics be a good exercise program for you? Yes ☐ No ☐
Explain.

Isotonic Exercises for Endurance and Mild Strengthening

Name_____ Section_____ Date_____

In addition to weight training there are other types of isotonic exercises that use gravity as the resistance. These can be modified to be suitable for those who are not able to lift heavy weights. These exercises can develop limited strength, but are primarily good for muscular endurance. They are frequently used for "figure development" by women, but are appropriate for anyone needing muscular endurance and limited strengthening, such as in postural correction.

Purpose

The purposes of this laboratory session are:

1. To give you an opportunity to experience gravity resisted exercises.
2. To familiarize you with exercises you may wish to include in your lifetime exercise program for muscular endurance, figure (physique) control, and posture correction.

Procedures

1. Read about the exercises on page 294.
2. Perform the exercises as described. Do ten repetitions of each exercise or as many as you can do in the time allotted by your instructor (see pages 295-298).

Results

Do you think you need to use any of these exercises? Yes ☐ No ☐ If so, which ones?

Conclusions and Implications

How would you use these exercises in your regular exercise program?

Flexibility Exercises

Name_____ Section_____ Date_____

Flexibility is not an aspect of health-related fitness that is built without effort. To attain flexibility it is necessary to stretch muscles regularly.

Purpose

The purposes of this laboratory session are:

1. To give you an opportunity to experience different flexibility exercises.
2. To acquaint you with a flexibility program that can be continued throughout your life.

Procedures

1. Read about the flexibility exercises on page 298.
2. Perform each of the exercises three times as described (on pages 299-301).

Results

Were you able to do all of the exercises? Yes ☐ No ☐
Were the exercises difficult? Yes ☐ No ☐
Could you tell which of your muscles were inflexible by performing the exercises? Yes ☐ No ☐ Which ones?

Conclusions and Implications

Will you choose any of these flexibility exercises for your lifetime program of exercise? Yes ☐ No ☐
If yes, which ones?

If no, why will you not use these exercises?

Sports for Physical Fitness

Name_____Section_____Date_____

Sports should be considered with the other types of exercise and physical activity programs as means for achieving health-related physical fitness. As noted in Concept 17, sports have various advantages and disadvantages as fitness programs. However, because there are so many different kinds of sports, it is really necessary to consider each sport individually when planning your exercise program. You should consider participation in the sport that is most likely to meet your own personal needs and interests.

Purpose

The purpose of this experiment is:

1. To explore the use of different sports as a part of your personal physical fitness program.

Procedures

1. On Chart 37.1 check those sports that you feel you might enjoy as a part of your regular exercise program.
2. On the same chart, rate your proficiency in each of the sports you checked in item 1 above. Use your own subjective rating (see scale below).

$$+ + + = \text{very high rating}$$
$$+ + = \text{good rating}$$
$$+ = \text{minimal rating}$$
$$- = \text{low rating}$$

3. Perform, in class or out, two or three different sports for thirty minutes to one hour each.
4. Assess the value of the sports you performed in terms of their worth (in your own opinion) for promoting various aspects of physical fitness. Make these ratings on Chart 37.1 using the rating scale in item 2 above.
5. Compare your ratings with the ratings of experts on page 249.

Chart 37.1 Physical Fitness Ratings for Sports*

Sport	Interest	Proficiency	Self-ratings			
			Cardiovascular Fitness	Muscular Endurance	Strength	Flexib
Bicycling	———	———	———	———	———	———
Swimming	———	———	———	———	———	———
Skating	———	———	———	———	———	———
Handball	———	———	———	———	———	———
Nordic Skiing	———	———	———	———	———	———
Alpine Skiing	———	———	———	———	———	———
Basketball	———	———	———	———	———	———
Tennis	———	———	———	———	———	———
Golf°°	———	———	———	———	———	———
Softball	———	———	———	———	———	———
Bowling	———	———	———	———	———	———

°Use the same rating scale as item 2 in the procedures to interpret expert ratings. E:
ratings are modified from those of seven physical fitness experts as presented in an ar
by Conrad, C. C. "How Different Sports Rate in Promoting Physical Fitness," *Me*
Times, 104:65-72, May 1972.
°°The experts based their rating of golf on the fact that some people use a cart or a ca

Results

List the names of the sports you chose on the blanks below. Summarize how your ratings compared with those of the experts concerning the values of each sport for developing physical fitness.

Sport ——————————————— . Summary of fitness values.

Sport ——————————————— . Summary of fitness values.

Sport ——————————————— . Summary of fitness values.

Control Weight	Expert Ratings				
	Cardiovascular Fitness	Muscular Endurance	Strength	Flexibility	Weight Control
———	+++	+++	++	+	+++
———	+++	+++	++	++	++
———	+++	+++	++	++	+++
———	+++	+++	++	++	+++
———	+++	+++	++	++	+++
———	++	+++	++	++	++
———	+++	+++	++	++	+++
———	++	++	++	++	++
———	+	+	+	+	−
———	−	+	−	+	−
———	−	−	−	+	−

Conclusions and Implications

Which sports do you feel you might actually include in your exercise program for a lifetime? Discuss.

Planning Your Personal Exercise Program

Name_____Section_____Date_____

It is hoped that every person will desire to develop and maintain physical fitness through exercise and activity. A physically *fit* person may be described as one who possesses the ability to work at peak efficiency in daily life and in any emergency situation that might arise. A fit person possesses buoyant health and performs well in the health-related aspects of physical fitness including endurance, strength, and flexibility. A fit person also possesses a relatively lean body and enough motor fitness to perform effectively in leisure-time pursuits.

Physical fitness is *not* the only important consideration in making decisions about future activities and exercise. A physically educated person is not only fit, but is one who can use his body effectively. He or she possesses efficient movement skills and is reasonably proficient in a variety of sports and other physical activities. The physically educated person also has a knowledge of and a desirable attitude toward exercise, sports, and dance.

It is one of the purposes of this book to present information that might contribute to the physical education of the reader. The measure of its success will be your decision to engage in adequate physical activity in the future.

Purpose

The purposes of this laboratory session are:

1. To plot a personal profile to be used in making decisions about future patterns of activity and exercise for YOU.
2. To develop your own personalized exercise program that can be continued for a lifetime.
3. To try out your personal exercise program.
4. To evaluate your personal exercise program to see if it meets the purposes for which it was intended.

Procedures

1. Plot your personal physical activity evaluation profile on Chart 38.1 (men) or Chart 38.2 (women). Circle the score you achieved on each of the tests taken during Labs 4 to 22.

2. Check your ratings on the various physical activity aspects in the appropriate boxes presented in the "results" section.
3. Using the information from items 1 and 2 above, PLAN A WEEKLY PROGRAM and record it on Chart 38.3. Include all of the exercises you feel you should do (including sports and games) on a regular basis to meet your physical activity needs. (Review Concept 19—Planning Your Exercise Program, pages 123-126).
4. Perform *one day's* activities from your exercise plan during class time. Ask your instructor for help if you have questions about your exercise plan.

Results

1. Circle your scores on Chart 38.1 (men) or Chart 38.2 (women).
2. Check the boxes that best reflect your performance!

	Attitude About Exercise	Strength & Muscular Endurance	Flexibility	Cardiovascular Fitness	Body Fatness	Posture, Feet, & Back	Skill-Related Fitness
Excellent	☐	☐	☐	☐	☐	☐	☐
Adequate for my needs	☐	☐	☐	☐	☐	☐	☐
Needs work	☐	☐	☐	☐	☐	☐	☐
Very poor	☐	☐	☐	☐	☐	☐	☐

3. Write in your exercise program on Chart 38.3.

Conclusions and Implications

Do you think you will perform your personal program regularly for the next year? Yes ☐ No ☐ Discuss.

Chart 38.1   Personal Evaluation Profile for Men

Very Poor	Poor	Marginal	Very Good	Excellent	Classification	
0-5	6-7	8-14	15-17	18	H F Scale	Attitude Scale First Test
0-5	6-7	8-14	15-17	18	Social	
0-5	6-7	8-14	15-17	18	Rec-Emot	
0-5	6-7	8-14	15-17	18	General	
0-20	21-31	32-56	57-68	69-72	Total	
0-5	6-7	8-14	15-17	18	H F Scale	Attitude Scale Second Test
0-5	6-7	8-14	15-17	18	Social	
0-5	6-7	8-14	15-17	18	Rec-Emot	
0-5	6-7	8-14	15-17	18	General	
0-21	21-31	32-56	57-68	69-72	Total	
0-3	4-5	6	7-8	9	Physical Fitness Test	
1.48—1.5	1.52-1.57	1.58-1.81	1.82-1.85	1.86	12 Minute Run	Cardiovascular Fitness
$\geq$ 121	120-111	110-91	90-80	$<$ 80	Step Test	
33	34-36	37-45	46-53	$\geq$ 54	Bicycle Test	
85	86-94	95-123	124-149	$>$ 150	Left Grip	Strength Tests
90	91-104	105-135	136-154	$>$ 155	Right Grip	
200	201-276	277-389	390-459	$>$ 460	Back Strength	
300	301-351	352-469	470-529	$\geq$ 530	Leg Strength	
675	676-825	826-1116	1117-1291	$>$ 1292	Total Strength	
4.80	4.81-5.20	5.21-7.09	7.10-7.49	$\geq$ 7.50	Strength Per/Lb/Wt	
0-5	6-10	11-22	23-30	$\geq$ 31	Sitting Tuck	Muscular Endurance
0-2	3-5	6-10	11-14	$\geq$ 15	Chins	
11	12-14	15-25	26-32	$\geq$ 33	Test I	Flexibility
0-3	4-5	6-11	12-16	$\geq$ 17	Test II	
-2	— 1-3	4-5	6	$>$ 7	Right Up Test III	
-5	— 4-3	— 2-3	4-5	$>$ 6	Left Up	
$\geq$ 20	18-19	15-17	11-14	0-10	% Fat	
$\geq$ 12	8-11	5-7	3-4	0-2	Posture	
10-12	7-9	4-6	1-3	0	Tension-Relaxation	
0-29	30-59	60-79	80-89	90-100	Balance	Motor Fitness Tests
$\geq$ 18.9	18.7-18.8	16.8-18.6	15.9-16.7	15.8	Agility	
5'9"	5'10"-6'3"	6'4"-7'8"	7'9"-8'5"	$\geq$ 8'6"	Power Jump	
0-2	3-4	5-10	11-13	14-15	Coordination	

Chart 38.2 Personal Evaluation Profile for Women

Very Poor	Poor	Marginal	Very Good	Excellent	Classification	
0-5	6-7	8-14	15-17	18	H F Scale	
0-5	6-7	8-14	15-17	18	Social	Attitude Scale First Test
0-5	6-7	8-14	15-17	18	Rec-Emot	
0-5	6-7	8-14	15-17	18	General	
0-20	21-31	32-56	57-68	69-72	Total	
0-5	6-7	8-14	15-17	18	H F Scale	
0-5	6-7	8-14	15-17	18	Social	Attitude Scale Second Test
0-5	6-7	8-14	15-17	18	Rec-Emot	
0-5	6-7	8-14	15-17	18	General	
0-20	21-31	32-56	57-68	69-72	Total	
0-3	4-5	6	7-8	9	Physical Fitness Test	
below .90	.90-1.09	1.10-1.30	1.40-1.49	1.5	12 Minute Run	
$\geqq$ 121	120-111	110-91	90-80	< 80	Step Test	Cardiovascular Fitness
29	30-35	36-41	42-46	$\geqq$ 47	Bicycle Test	
39	40-47	48-75	76-81	$\geqq$ 82	Left Grip	
48	49-55	56-82	83-89	$\geqq$ 90	Right Grip	
85	86-114	115-214	215-244	$\geqq$ 245	Back Strength	
85	86-114	145-249	250-299	$\geqq$ 300	Leg Strength	Strength Tests
257	258-360	361-620	621-713	$\geqq$ 714	Total Strength	
2.00	2.10-2.89	2.90-4.79	4.80-5.49	$\geqq$ 5.50	Strength Per/Lb/Wt	
0-2	3-6	7-14	15-20	$\geqq$ 21	Sitting Tuck	Muscular Endurance
0			1	2	Chins	
11	12-14	15-21	22-27	$\geqq$ 28	Test I	
0-3	4-5	6-12	13-16	$\geqq$ 17	Test II	Flexibility
-2	— 1-3	4-6	7	> 8	Right Up Test III	
4	— 3-0	1-5	6-7	> 8	Left Up	
$\geqq$ 28	23-27	18-22	13-17	0-12	% Fat	
$\geqq$ 12	8-11	5-7	3-4	0-2	Posture	
10-12	8-11	4-6	1-3	0	Tension-Relaxation	
0-29	30-59	60-79	80-89	90-100	Balance	
$\geqq$ 23.5	22.4-23.4	18.7-22.3	17.5-18.6	17.4	Agility	Motor Fitness Tests
4'1"	4'2"-4'7"	4'8"-5'9"	5'10"-6'7"	$\geqq$ 6'8"	Power Jump	
0-1	2-3	4-9	10-12	13-15	Coordination	

Chart 38.3 Personal Exercise Program (Regular Weekly Schedule)

REASON FOR EXERCISES CHOSEN

	Endurance (Cardiovascular Fitness)	Strength	Muscular Endurance	Flexibility	Weight Control	Skill-Related Fitness
Monday						
Tuesday						
Wednesday						
Thursday						
Friday						
Saturday						
Sunday						

List the specific exercises, sports, or activities you would do for each specific purpose. If you would not exercise daily do not write in blanks under these days.

Physical Activity for a Lifetime

Name_____Section_____Date_____

As the typical American grows older his or her physical fitness tends to decline. At least one study indicates that the health-related physical fitness of the average American woman begins to decline in the early teens and begins in the average American man in the late teens. This decline is in spite of the fact that our greatest potential for fitness is between ages twenty-five and thirty.

Much of the decrease in physical and mental function that accompanies aging is a result of disuse rather than age. We are all capable of considerably more physical fitness later in life than is characterized by the typical American.

Purpose

The purposes of the laboratory session are:

1. To estimate your fitness needs at age forty.
2. To plan a program for yourself at age forty.
3. To determine the difference in exertion for your current program and your program for later life.

Procedures

1. Assume that your age is forty (or the age of a parent or relative near that age). Look up your cardiovascular threshold of training for the appropriate age. Guess your resting heart rate (it tends to go up as you get older and less fit). Record it in the "results" section.
2. Estimate what exercise would make you reach the cardiovascular threshold of training for a person near forty. (Make this determination on the basis of how fit you expect to be at forty or how fit the person is whose age you are assuming.) Write this exercise down in the results section and note the rate (e.g., one mile in seven minutes).
3. List three flexibility exercises and three strength or muscular endurance exercises that you think you should be performing (list only those you really think you could do at that age). Record in results section.

4. Perform the cardiovascular exercise for fifteen minutes and do the flexibility and strength-muscular endurance exercises.

Results

What will your cardiovascular threshold of training be at age forty?
96/120 bpm   96 – 120

What exercise would you do to get the heart rate to the level noted above for age forty? _____ _____

                               exercise   rate (if running how fast)

List three flexibility exercises you would do at age forty.

	Exercise	Repetitions
1.	_____	_____
2.	_____	_____
3.	_____	_____

List three strength or muscular endurance exercises you would do at age forty.

	Exercise	Repetitions
1.	_____	_____
2.	_____	_____
3.	_____	_____

How much easier for you were these exercises than your own program?

Do you really think you will be fit enough to do the above listed exercises at age forty?

Could your parent of the same sex or a relative of about forty do the exercises you have selected? Yes ☐ No ☐ Why or why not?

At age forty do you expect to be fitter or less fit than the typical person your age? Fitter ☐ Average ☐ Less Fit ☐ Explain.

Could you help a person forty or over plan an exercise program? Yes ☐ No ☐ Explain.

Reassessing the Values of Physical Activity

Name_____ Section_____ Date_____

In Laboratory 1, an assessment was made of your personal feelings about physical activity. Before making a decision concerning future exercise and physical activity habits, a reassessment might be helpful.

Purpose

The purpose of this laboratory session is to help you to detect any change in attitude that may have occurred during the course of this class.

Procedures

Read each of the sixteen items on page 263 and answer them either as "strongly agree," "agree," "undecided," "disagree," or "strongly disagree." Give the answer that best indicates the way *YOU* feel. Try not to use the response "undecided" unless absolutely necessary. Do not look at your first test. Score the sixteen items using the scoring method on page 264.

Expected Results

Do you think your attitude test scores will be different from your scores the first time you took the test? Yes ☐ No ☐
Check the changes that you think have occurred.

	same	higher	lower
Health and Fitness	☐	☐	☐
Social Scale	☐	☐	☐
Relaxation	☐	☐	☐
General	☐	☐	☐
Total Test	☐	☐	☐

Results

After scoring your test write your rating on each scale of the attitude test below and note whether your score increased or decreased.

	Rating Test 1	Rating Test 2	+	same	—
Health and Physical Fitness Scale					
Social Scale					
Recreational-Emotional Release Scale					
General Attitude Scale					
Test Total					

Conclusions and Implications

Do you think the sixteen-item test could detect accurately changes in your attitude? Yes ☐ No ☐ Explain.

What is your attitude about physical activity at this time?

Attitude Test

Strongly Agree	Agree	Unde-cided	Dis-agree	Strongly Disagree		SCORE
☐	☐	☐	☐	☐	1. Physical education is all right for those who like sports but is not for me.	____
☐	☐	☐	☐	☐	2. Physical exercise and activity are as dangerous to health as they are valuable.	____
☐	☐	☐	☐	☐	3. I enjoy taking part in a sport just to get away from it all.	____
☐	☐	☐	☐	☐	4. I like to participate best in those games that involve working as a team.	____
☐	☐	☐	☐	☐	5. Physical activity is one way to rid yourself of the worries and tensions of everyday life.	____
☐	☐	☐	☐	☐	6. Probably one of the main values of sports is to fill leisure time in our automated society.	____
☐	☐	☐	☐	☐	7. I would only enroll in physical education if it were a graduation requirement.	____
☐	☐	☐	☐	☐	8. The time some people spend exercising could probably be better spent in other ways.	____
☐	☐	☐	☐	☐	9. Sports and games build social confidence.	____
☐	☐	☐	☐	☐	10. Industry might be wise to substitute exercise breaks for coffee breaks.	____
☐	☐	☐	☐	☐	11. Competition in sports is often a way to destroy good friendships.	____
☐	☐	☐	☐	☐	12. Most jobs provide all the exercise and activity a person needs.	____
☐	☐	☐	☐	☐	13. Everyone should have skill in several sports that can be used later in life.	____
☐	☐	☐	☐	☐	14. Social dancing and other similar forms of activity are a waste of time.	____
☐	☐	☐	☐	☐	15. Health and physical fitness are basic to all of life's activities.	____
☐	☐	☐	☐	☐	16. I would recommend that everyone take physical education because of the important nature of the subject.	____

Score the attitude test as follows:

1. For items 1, 2, 7, 8, 11, 12, and 14 give one point for Strongly Agree, two for Agree, three for Undecided, four for Disagree, and five for Strongly Disagree. Put the correct number on the blank to the right of these statements.
2. For items 3, 4, 5, 6, 9, 10, 13, 15, and 16 give five points for Strongly Agree, four for Agree, three for Undecided, two for Disagree, and one for Strongly Disagree. Put the correct number on the blank to the right of these statements.
3. Add the scores for items 2, 8, 12, and 15. This total represents your health and fitness attitude score.
4. Add the scores for items 4, 9, 11, and 14. This total represents your social attitude score.
5. Add the scores for items 3, 5, 6, and 13. This total represents your recreational-emotional attitude score.
6. Add the scores for items 1, 7, 10, and 16. This total represents your general attitude score.
7. Circle your scores on the chart given and record them on page 262.

Attitude Rating Scale

	Attitude Scale First Test					Attitude Scale Second Test				
	HF Scale	Social	Rec-Emot	General	Total	HF Scale	Social	Rec-Emot	General	Total
Excellent (Ex)		18	18	18	69-72	18	18	18	18	69-72
Good	15-17	15-17	15-17	15-17	57-68	15-17	15-17	15-17	15-17	57-68
Marginal (M)	8-14	8-14	8-14	8-14	32-56	8-14	8-14	8-14	8-14	32-56
Poor	6-7	6-7	6-7	6-7	21-31	6-7	6-7	6-7	6-7	21-31
Very Poor (VP)	0-5	0-5	0-5	0-5	0-20	0-5	0-5	0-5	0-5	0-20

8. Record your results by circling the appropriate score above. Determine your rating for each scale and record it in the results section.

Appendixes

The treatment for painful spines ranges from surgical fusion to more conservative measures such as procain injections, muscle relaxant pills, ethyl chloride spray, traction, bed rest, heat, massage, and therapeutic exercise. Exercise is not a cure-all and should not be used indiscriminately for backaches. If a doctor recommends exercise for the back, or if an individual is susceptible to back strain and/or simply wishes to prevent its occurrence, then be assured, proper exercise will be invaluable.

The exercises presented here are preventive and remedial exercises for the back. Some are designed primarily to strengthen the abdominals and to stretch the lumbar muscles; others are designed to strengthen back muscles. Omitted from this series of exercises are those that stretch shortened hip flexors. If it is determined that you need to stretch the iliopsoas muscles, consult your instructor. If you have had surgery or an injury, you should wait until your physician advises you to start exercising. If you have been inactive for a period of time, it would be wise to perform these exercises for several days before tackling a job that might strain your back. Start slowly and gradually increase the number of repetitions; perform the exercises three times daily for maximum benefits. If soreness occurs the next day, reduce the frequency until strength is increased and soreness ceases to occur.

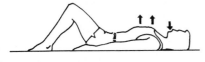

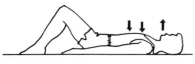

1. **Deep Breathing.** In the hook-lying position, with arms at sides, take a deep breath, expanding the chest as much as possible; exhale slowly, allowing the chest to return to its normal position. Keep the back and neck flat. Repeat very slowly five or six times. (mild back stretcher)

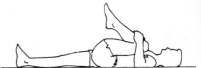

2. **Alternate Knee-to-Chest.** In the hook-lying position, draw one knee up to the chest and pull it down tightly with the hands, then slowly return to the original position. Repeat with the other knee. Repeat with each leg ten to twenty times. (stretches lumbar muscles)

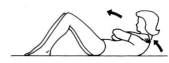

3. **Trunk Curl.** Lie on the back with the knees bent. Roll the head and neck forward, then the shoulders. Roll as far forward as possible without lifting the lower back off the floor. Hold. Return to start and repeat. (strengthens abdominals)

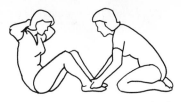

4. Bent Knee Sit-up. Lie on the back with knees bent. Roll the head, neck, and shoulders forward in sequence. Lift the back off the floor. Return to starting position and repeat. Feet may be held. Arms may be placed at the sides, across the chest or behind the head. (strengthens abdominals)

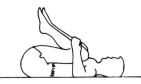

5. Double Knee-to-Chest. In the hook-lying position, draw both knees to the chest and pull them down tight against the chest with the arms. Hold this position for twenty-five seconds. Return to starting position and repeat five or six times. Before raising the knees tighten the abdominal muscles and hold the back flat. (stretches lumbar muscles)

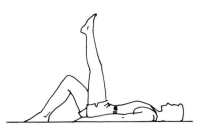

6. Alternate Leg Extension. In the hook-lying position, draw one knee to the chest, then extend the knee and point the foot toward the ceiling. Return to the starting position by drawing the knee back to the chest before sliding the foot to the floor. Repeat with other leg. Repeat cycle four or five times. (stretches lumbar muscles)

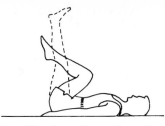

7. Double Leg Extension. In the hook-lying position, draw both knees to the chest, then extend both legs toward the ceiling, keeping the lower back flat. Return to the starting position by drawing the knees to the chest before placing the feet on the floor. Repeat three or four times. (stretches lumbar muscles) (*Note*: This is a more strenuous exercise and the weak person should not attempt it until the other exercises have been performed three or four weeks.)

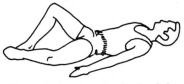

8. Knee Abduction. In the hook-lying position, let the knees fall apart alternately, right and left as far as they will go, thirty or forty times. (stretches hip flexors and adductors)

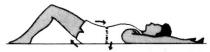

9. Isometric Contractions. In the hook-lying position, tighten the abdominal muscles and try to flatten the lower back against the floor. At the same time, tighten the hip and thigh muscles. Hold the contractions for six seconds, then relax. Repeat five or six times. Breathe normally during the contraction—do not hold the breath. (strengthens abdominals)

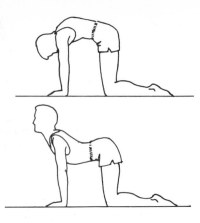

10. **Cat Backs.** Kneel on all fours. Contract the abdominals strongly, tilting the pelvis backward and making the back hump upward while dropping the head. Hold the rounded back position for six seconds and then relax, letting the back sway and abdomen sag as the head is lifted. Repeat five or six times. (strengthens abdominals)

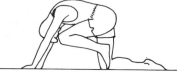

11. **Knee-to-Nose Touch.** Kneel on all fours. Drop the head and try to touch the nose with one knee. Then extend that leg backward parallel with the floor (avoid arching the back). Return to the starting position. Alternate legs ten to twenty times. (stretches lumbar muscles and strengthens gluteals)

B. The following exercises are designed to strengthen the back muscles:

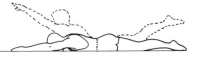

1. For those who do **NOT** have weak abdominals and/or lordosis:

Prone Arm and Leg Lift. Lie prone with the arms extended in front of the head. Raise: (a) the right arm toward the ceiling and return; (b) the left arm and return; (c) both arms and return; (d) repeat with legs—right, left and both; (e) try right arm and right leg; (f) left arm and left leg; (g) right arm and left leg; (h) left arm and right leg; and (i) both arms and both legs. (strengthens upper and lower back and hip extensors)

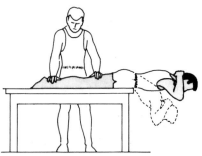

2. For those WITH weak abdominals and/or lordosis:

a. **Upper Trunk Lift.** Lie on table or bench with upper half of body hanging over the edge. Have a partner stabilize the feet while the trunk is raised parallel to the floor. Start with the hands under the thighs; as strength develops, place hands behind neck. Do not raise past the horizontal or arch the back. (strengthens upper back)

Tension Relieving Exercises

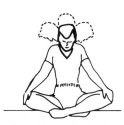

1. Head Circle. Roll the head slowly in a large circle first clockwise and then counterclockwise. Close your eyes and let your mouth fall open during the exercise. Repeat several times.

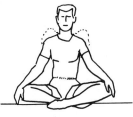

2. Shoulder Lift. Hunch the shoulders as high as possible and then let them drop. Repeat several times. Inhale on the lift; exhale on the drop.

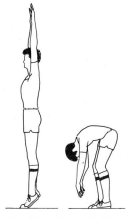

3. Trunk Stretch and Drop. Stand and reach as high as possible; tiptoe

and stretch every muscle, then collapse completely, letting knees flex and trunk, head, and arms dangle (see Trunk Swing Illustration). Repeat two or three times.

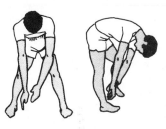

4. Trunk Swings. Following the trunk drop (described above), bounce gently with a minimum of muscular effort. Set the trunk swinging from side to side by shifting the weight from one foot to the other, letting the heels come off the floor alternately. Then with a slight springing movement of the lower back, gently bob up and down, keeping the entire body (especially the neck) limp.

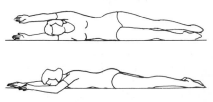

5. Tension Contrast. With arms extended overhead, lie on your side; tense the body as "stiff as a board," then "let go" and relax letting the body fall either forward or backward in whatever direction it loses balance. Continue "letting go" for a few seconds after falling and feel like you are still "sinking." Repeat on the other side.

A³ The Aerobics Program

To achieve the benefits of the Aerobics Program, an individual should exercise a minimum of three times a week and earn at least thirty points a week from the chart below. At first you may wish to begin by earning ten to fifteen points a week and then work up to thirty.

Aerobics Point Chart*

Points	Walking-Running (Time for 1 Mile)	Cycling (Speed for 2 Miles)	Swimming (300 yds.)	Handball Basket-ball	Stationary Running for 5 Min.	Stationary Running for 10 Min.	Points
0	Over 20 Min.	Less than 10 MPH	Over 10 Min.	Less than 10 Min.	Less than 60 Steps/min.	Less than 50 Steps/min.	0
1	20:00-14:30 Min.	10-15 MPH	8:00-10:00 Min.	10 Min.	60-70 Steps/min.	50-65 Steps/min.	1
2	14:29-12:00 Min.	15-20 MPH	7:30-8:00 Min.	20 Min.	80-90 Steps/min.	65-70 Steps/min.	2
3	11:59-10:00 Min.	Over 20 MPH	6:00-7:30 Min.	30 Min.		70-80 Steps/min.	3
4	9:59-8:00 Min.			40 Min.		80-90 Steps/min.	4
5	7:59-6:30 Min.			50 Min.			5
6	Less than 6:30 Min.			60 Min.			6

*Used by permission of K. Cooper, *The New Aerobics* (New York: M. Evans and Co., 1970.)

If you plan to use the Aerobics Program as part of your regular exercise plan you should read: *The New Aerobics* (58) and *Aerobics for Women* (57).

Aerobic Dance is a modification of Aerobics that has gained much popularity recently. It combines aerobic exercise with dance to provide many exercise benefits. The interested person is referred to Concept 17.

Advantages and Disadvantages of the Aerobics Program

Advantages	*Disadvantages*
1. Develops cardiovascular fitness.	1. Is principally a cardiovascular fitness program which would have to be supplemented with exercises for other aspects of health-related fitness.
2. Provides a program with a variety of activities.	
3. Provides a method of evaluating progress (12-minute run).	2. Because of individual differences points may vary for activities from individual to individual. (see Ref. no. 58)

The Adult Fitness Program of Exercise

The adult physical fitness program as developed by the President's Council on Sports and Physical Fitness is designed as a total program of exercise. A manual is available that includes exercises graduated in intensity from easy to very difficult depending on the needs of the person. As you perform one set of exercises for a period of time and they become easy, you then progress to the next set of exercises. The following is a *sample* program that is presented to give you an idea of the nature of the Adult Fitness Program. If you choose to perform these activities you should read the *Adult Fitness Manual* (219).

Advantages and Disadvantages of the Adult Fitness Program

Advantages	*Disadvantages*
1. Graduated in intensity to meet the needs of a wide variety of people.	1. Because it is basically a calisthenics program it may be difficult to sustain interest in the program over a long period of time.
2. Develops most all aspects of health-related fitness though it is doubtful that the program would build cardiovascular fitness for all people.	2. Would need to be supplemented with cardiovascular fitness exercise for many.

Adult Physical Fitness Exercises

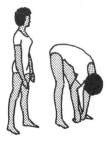 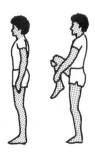

1. **Bend and Stretch.** Starting position: Stand erect, feet shoulder-width apart.
Action: Count 1. Bend trunk forward and down, flexing knees. Stretch gently in attempt to touch fingers to toes or floor. Count 2. Return to starting position.
Note: Do slowly, stretch and relax at intervals rather than in rhythm.

2. **Knee Lift.** Starting position: Stand erect, feet together, arms at sides.
Action: Count 1. Raise left knee as high as possible, grasping leg with hands and pulling knee against body while keeping back straight. Count 2. Lower to starting position. Counts 3 and 4. Repeat with right knee.

ORIENTATION PROGRAM*   **GOAL**

Conditioning exercises	Repetitions
1. Bend and stretch	10
2. Knee lift	10 left, 10 right
3. Wing stretcher	20
4. Half knee bend	10
5. Arm circles	15 each way
6. Body bender	10 left, 10 right
7. Prone arch	10
8. Knee push-up	6
9. Head and shoulder curl	5
10. Ankle stretch	15

Circulatory activity (choose one each workout)
Walking ....½ mile
Rope (skip 15 sec.; rest 60 sec.) ....3 series

Note: Exercises 1 and 7 are not recommended for those experiencing low back difficulties.

*Used by permission President's Council on Physical Fitness and Sports. *Adult Physical Fitness.* Washington, D. C.

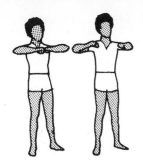

3. Wing Stretcher. Starting position: Stand erect, elbows at shoulder height, fists clenched in front of chest.
Action: Count 1. Thrust elbows backward vigorously without arching back. Keep head erect, elbows at shoulder height. Count 2. Return to starting position.

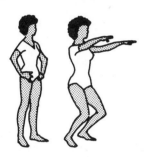

4. Half Knee Bend. Starting position: Stand erect, hands on hips.
Action: Count 1. Bend knees halfway while extending arms forward, palms down. Count 2. Return to starting position.

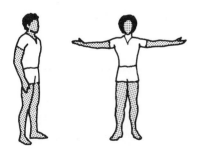

5. Arm Circles. Starting position: Stand erect, arms extended sideward at shoulder height, palms up.

Action: Describe small circles backward with hands. Keep head erect. Do 15 backward circles. Reverse, turn palms down and do 15 small circles forward.

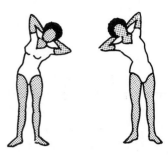

6. Body Bender. Starting position: Stand, feet shoulder-width apart, hands behind neck, fingers interlaced.
Action: Count 1. Bend trunk sideward to left as far as possible, keeping hands behind neck. Count 2. Return to starting position. Counts 3 and 4. Repeat to the right.

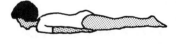

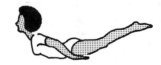

7. Prone Arch. Starting position: Lie face down, hands tucked under thighs. Action: Count 1. Raise head, shoulders and legs from floor. Count 2. Return to starting position.

Circulatory Activities

WALKING—Step off at a lively pace, swing arms and breathe deeply. *ROPE*—Any form of skipping or jumping is acceptable. Gradually increase the tempo as your skill and condition improve.

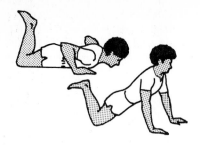

Action: Count 1. Tighten abdominal muscles, lift head and pull shoulders and elbows off floor. Hold for four seconds. Count 2. Return to starting position.

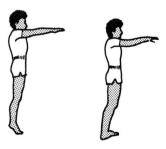

8. **Knee Push-up.** Starting position: Lie on floor, face down, legs together, knees bent with feet raised off floor, hands on floor under shoulders, palms down.

Action: Count 1. Push upper body off floor until arms are fully extended and body is in straight line from head to knees. Count 2. Return to starting position.

10. **Ankle Stretch.** Starting position: Stand on a stair, large book, or block of wood, with weight on balls of feet and heels raised.

Action: Count 1. Lower heels. Count 2. Raise heels.

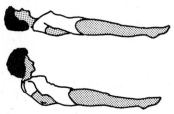

9. **Head and Shoulder Curl.** Starting position: Lie on back, hands tucked under small of back, palms down.

⁵ The Canadian XBX and 5BX Programs

The Canadian Air Force Program consists of two separate parts: 5BX for men and XBX for women. These graduated programs are arranged so that a specific number of exercises and repetitions are performed, depending upon your initial fitness. The more fit people select exercises from a chart listing more difficult exercises while the less fit people select exercises from a chart illustrating less difficult exercises.

The XBX plan contains four charts of ten exercises, with each chart more difficult than the preceding one. Each chart is divided into twelve fitness levels. The 5BX includes six charts of five exercises each with each chart divided into twelve fitness "levels." Intensity of exercise increases progressively as one moves from level to level and from chart to chart. Persons planning to use the program should obtain a copy of the book. A sample program of moderate intensity is presented below.* The program is selected from the XBX plan for women, but is very similar to the plan for men.

Sample Program	Number of Repetitions
Exercise 1	10
Exercise 2	16
Exercise 3	12
Exercise 4	24
Exercise 5**	26
Exercise 6	28
Exercise 7	28
Exercise 8	22
Exercise 9	8
Exercise 10	140

*Used by permission Royal Canadian Air Force, *Exercise Plans for Physical Fitness.* Queen's Printer, Ottawa, Canada: Revised U.S. Edition, 1962. By special arrangement with *This Week Magazine.*

**Exercises with double asterisks have been modified to avoid possible back problems for those with weak back muscles.

Advantages and Disadvantages of the XBX and 5BX Programs

Advantages

1. Develops most all aspects of health-related fitness though it is doubtful that the program would build cardiovascular fitness in many people.

2. Graduated in intensity to meet the needs of a wide variety of people.

Disadvantages

1. Would need to be supplemented with cardiovascular fitness exercise for many.

2. Because it is basically a calisthenics program it may be difficult to sustain interest in the program over a long period of time.

XBX and 5BX Exercises

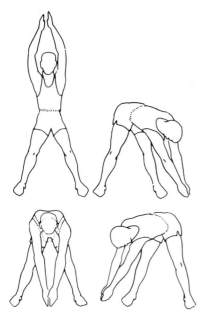

knee as high as possible, grasping knee and shin with hands. Pull leg against body. Keep straight throughout. Lower foot to floor. Repeat with right leg. Continue by alternating legs.

Count. Left knee raise plus right knee raise counts as one repetition.

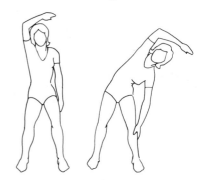

1. **Toe Touching.** Start. Stand erect, feet about sixteen inches apart, arms over head. Bend down to touch floor outside left foot. Bob up and down to touch floor between feet. Bob again and bend to touch floor outside right foot. Return to starting position.

Count. Each return to the starting position counts one repetition.

3. **Lateral Bending.** Start. Stand erect, feet twelve inches apart, right arm extended over head, bent at elbow. Keeping back straight, bend sidewards from waist to left. Slide left hand down leg as far as possible, at the same time press to left with right arm. Return to starting position and change arm positions. Repeat to right. Continue by alternating to left then right.

Count. Bend to left plus bend to right counts as one repetition.

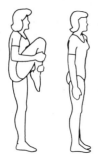

2. **Knee Raising.** Start. Stand erect, feet together, arms at sides. Raise left

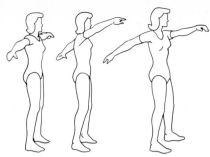

4. **Arm Circling.** Start. Stand erect, feet twelve inches apart, arms at sides. Make large circles with arms in a windmill action—one arm following other and both moving at same time. Do half the number of repetitions making backward circles and half making forward circles.
Count. Each full circle by both arms counts as one repetition.

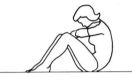

5. **Sit-ups.** ** Start. Lie on back, knees bent and together, arms across chest. Roll shoulders and trunk forward, move to a sitting position. Return to starting position.
Count. Each return to the starting position counts as one repetition.

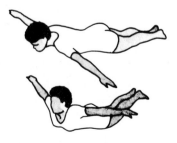

6. **Chest and Leg Raising.** Start. Lie face down, legs straight and together, arms stretched sidewards at shoulder level. Raise entire upper body and both legs from floor as high as possible. Keep legs straight. Return to starting position.

Count. Each return to the starting position counts as one repetition.

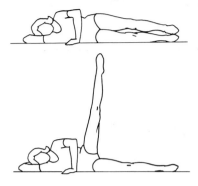

7. **Side Leg Raising.** Start. Lie on side with the legs straight along floor, top arm used for balance. Raise upper leg until it is perpendicular to floor. Lower to starting position.
Count. Each leg raise counts one. Do half the number of repetitions raising left leg. Roll to other side and do half with the right leg.

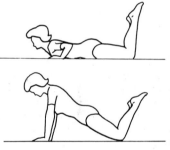

8. **Modified Push-up.** Start. Lie face down, hands directly under shoulders, knees on the floor. Raise body from floor by straightening it from head to knees. In the "up" position, the body should be in a straight line and elbows, forearms, and feet in contact with floor. Lower to starting position. Keep head up throughout.
Count. Each return to the starting position counts as one repetition.

Appendixes

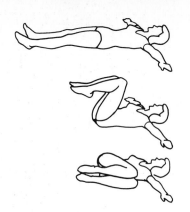

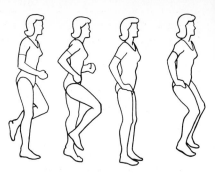

9. **Leg-overs—Tuck.** Start. Lie on back, legs straight and together, arms stretched sidewards at shoulder level, palms down. Raise both legs from floor, bending at hips and knees until in a tuck position. Lower legs to left, keeping knees together and both shoulders on floor. Twist hips and lower legs to floor on right side. Twist hips to tuck position and return to starting position. Keep knees close to abdomen throughout.

Count. Each return to the starting position counts as one repetition.

10. **Run and Half Knee Bends.** Start. Stand erect, feet together, arms at sides. Starting with left leg, run in place raising feet at least six inches from floor.

Count. Each time the left foot touches the floor counts as one repetition. After each fifty counts do ten half knee bends.

Half Knee Bends. Start with hands on hips, feet together, body erect. Bend at knees and hips, lowering body until thigh and calf form an angle of about 110 degrees. Do not bend knees past a right angle. Keep back straight. Return to starting position.

$\mathbf{A}^6$ The Progressive Rhythmical Endurance Program

1. Depending upon your physical fitness test scores, you should participate for five, ten, or fifteen minutes. As you become more fit, you should progress to the point where you can exercise continuously for at least fifteen minutes. All persons should begin with the stretching exercises listed below.

2. Exercise should be done continuously. As you finish a specific exercise, get up and jog in place or jog in a circle.

3. After progressing to the point where you can exercise for the full fifteen minutes, you should begin jogging after completing all of the exercises. Some participants progress to the point where they perform the fifteen minutes of exercise and jog for an additional five to twenty minutes.

Advantages and Disadvantages of Progressive Rhythmical Endurance Exercises

Advantages

1. Develops all health-related aspects of fitness.

2. Can be kept interesting by changing the different exercises periodically.

Disadvantages

1. Is best when done with a group. Interest may lag if you must exercise by yourself.

A Sample Program*

Stretching	5-Minute Circle Exercises	10-Minute Circle Exercises	15-Minute Circle Exercises
All stretching is passive and each exercise is held 5 to 6 seconds	jog in a circle 1 minute	15 jumping jacks	jog in a circle
3 standing hamstring stretches	7 bent knee sit-ups	7 knee touches	10 knee dips with each leg
3 lateral trunk stretches	lateral shuffle in circle	15 jumping jacks	jog in a circle
3 sitting trunk stretches	10 side leg-lifts (each leg)	jog in a circle	5 bent knee sit-ups
3 back hyper-extensions	25 side hop-kicks	5 bent-knee sit-ups	5 lateral leg-lifts (each leg)
	10 back leg-lifts (one leg at a time)	jog in a circle backward	5 interval sprints (first jog a lap, walk a lap)
	jog in a circle	7 push-ups	
		5 long stride steps with each leg	
		jog in a circle	

*Adapted from an article by C. B. Corbin, "An Exercise Program for Large Groups," *The Physical Educator* 30:46-47, March 1973. Used by permission.

Some of the exercises are illustrated below:

Standing Hamstring Stretchers

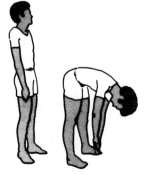

Lateral Trunk Stretchers

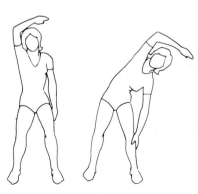

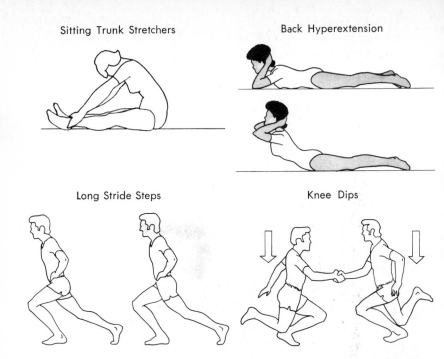

Sitting Trunk Stretchers

Back Hyperextension

Long Stride Steps

Knee Dips

Some general suggestions for using this exercise program are:

1. Stretch first to establish a pattern of regular stretching and to help eliminate possible soreness associated with the regular exercise program.
2. Start "too easy" rather than "too hard." You can always increase intensity after you determine your reaction to the exercise. You may wish to start out exercising for five or ten minutes and gradually progress to fifteen minutes.
3. If you exercise in a group you may want to select a daily leader to choose the exercises. This can help motivate group members.
4. Vary the exercises daily but make sure all body parts are exercised.
5. Walk outside the circle if you find you need a slower pace. If the exercises are too difficult, start with what you can handle, but try to exercise continuously even if it is just walking at first.
6. Use whatever exercises are appropriate for your individual needs. The ones listed are merely suggestions.

 A⁷   **The Circuit Training Program**

A Circuit Training program can involve six to ten different exercise stations. Each of the stations should require you to perform a different exercise for a different aspect of fitness and for different muscles. Be careful not to plan two stations in a row that require the use of the same muscles.

This is a *sample program* to familiarize you with the concept of Circuit Training. You can develop your own program using exercises at each station designed to meet your own exercise needs.

You may begin at any station. Perform the exercise at each station within a three-minute time period. Some may wish to perform as many exercises as possible in three minutes before going to the next station. Continue until you have completed the entire circuit.

Advantages and Disadvantages of the Circuit Training Program

Advantages

1. A wide variety of exercises can be used to maintain interest.

2. It is a good type of program for use with groups.

3. For some it provides incentive. You can keep records of performance and try to improve on your previous performance.

Disadvantages

1. This type of program would have to be done continually if it is to develop cardiovascular fitness.

2. May require more space and equipment than are available.

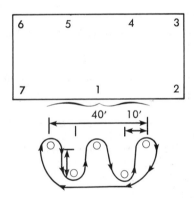

1. Agility Run—Put markers as indicated in the diagram. Begin at any place and run around the markers ten times within a three-minute time span. (You may wish to run the course as many times as you can in three minutes after you have been exercising regularly for a period of time.)

2. Chins—Grasp a bar with the palms facing away from the body. Do three chins. Repeat three times within three minutes. (You may wish to do as many chins as you can within the three-minute period.)

3. Step Up—Step up and down (right foot up, left foot up, right foot down, left foot down) on a bench fifteen to twenty inches high. Do fifty steps in three minutes. (You may wish to do as many steps as you can in the three-minute period.)

4. Shoulder Curls—Lie on the floor with the knees bent at about 90 degrees (feet on floor). Curl the chin, head, and shoulders forward as far as possible

without lifting the lower back off the floor. Repeat seven curls three different times in the three-minute period. (You may wish to do as many curls as possible in the three-minute period.)

5. Trunk Lift—Lie prone on a bench or table with the legs hanging over the edge. Raise the legs parallel to the floor and lower them. Repeat seven lifts three different times in three minutes. (You may wish to do as many lifts as possible in the three-minute period.)

6. Jump Rope—Jump rope for thirty seconds, rest for thirty seconds. Repeat for three minutes. (You may wish to jump for the full three minutes and to count the number of jumps completed in the three-minute period.)

7. Floor reach—Stand with the feet apart and the legs nearly straight. Bend forward at the hips and reach down and through the legs. Reach to a spot on the floor as far behind you as possible. Hold for eight seconds. Repeat five times in three minutes.

"Speed Play" or Fartlek Exercise

Speed Play (originally called Fartlek, the Swedish word for speed play) features varied speed running, walking, and some calisthenics. The program is designed to be psychologically stimulating by introducing a change in scenery and changing the pace of running. Those who prefer this type of running feel that it offers more diversity than jogging. Ideally, Speed Play is done over a course that provides a variety of terrain as opposed to being performed on a track. It can, however, be done on a track.

Advantages and Disadvantages of Speed Play or Fartlek Exercise

Advantages	*Disadvantages*
1. A good means of achieving cardiovascular fitness and, to a lesser extent, other health-related fitness aspects.	1. The fast "anaerobic" sprints may be inappropriate for beginners and some older runners.
2. Psychologically stimulating because of the break in monotony from changing speeds and scenery.	2. Primarily a cardiovascular program.
	3. You must have more than a little information to plan a good speed play program of the appropriate intensity.

You can plan your own Speed Play program using your own course that may include up and downhill running (common in the foothills of Sweden where it was developed) and other variations. The following is a sample program of moderate intensity.

The Program (A Sample)*

1. Jog easily for three minutes.
2. Perform brisk calisthenics—no rest between exercises.
   a. Trunk stretch—With the feet spread, reach through the legs as far as possible. Hold for eight seconds. Repeat three times. (See page 279.)
   b. Do five to ten bent knee sit-ups. (See page 277.)
   c. Run in place for fifty steps.
   d. Do five to ten push-ups or modified push-ups. (See page 295.)
   e. Do ten side leg raises with each leg. (See page 277.)
3. Run 200 yards at ¾ speed. Run on grassy area if possible.
4. Walk 200 yards.
5. Repeat 3 and 4.
6. Jog for two minutes.
7. Run 100 yards at ¾ speed.
8. Walk 100 yards.
9. Repeat 7 and 8.
10. Jog two minutes.

*If this *sample* program is too vigorous for your current level of fitness, walk instead of performing the exercise as outlined.

Interval Training

Interval Training is a type of anaerobic exercise that involves alternate running and resting. Interval Training is considered to be intermittent exercise and to be effective one should use the Threshold of Training Guidelines discussed in the section on Cardiovascular Fitness on pages 17-18.

Advantages and Disadvantages of Interval Training

Advantages	Disadvantages
1. Anaerobic or interval exercise is a good method of building cardiovascular fitness.	1. Interval sprints may be inappropriate for beginners and some older people.
2. Proponents argue that alternate running and walking is more interesting than the more regular nature of jogging.	2. Interval training is designed primarily as a cardiovascular fitness program.
3. If planned properly you can do more work for improving fitness in a shorter period of time.	

For longer distances (more than 100 yards) running should be estimated at approximately eighty percent of your maximum running speed. Rest periods for these longer runs should be of the same length as the running and should not be complete rests but should consist of walking or slow jogging. Shorter runs may be done above eighty percent of maximum speed. Rests should end when the heart rate returns to 120.

The Program (A Sample)

1. Jog for three minutes to get warmed up.
2. Run for 440 yards around a track or elsewhere at eighty percent of maximum speed.
3. Walk 220 yards.
4. Repeat 2 and 3.
5. Run 100 yards at 80 percent effort or faster. Immediately after exercise count your ten-second heart rate. Continue to count the heart rate for ten-second intervals until the heart rate for one ten-second period is 120 or less. Then repeat the 100-yard run.
6. Do five 100-yard runs with alternate rests. Walk or slow jog during rests. (If no watch or clock is available, walk for about 100 yards or jog about 150 yards between runs). If you plan to use interval running regularly you should get a watch and determine accurately the length of your rest period.
7. Repeat steps 2 and 3.

 Jogging

Jogging is a type of slow running that can be used to improve your level of cardiovascular fitness. To be effective you should jog fast enough to elevate your heart rate to the Threshold of Training. To determine your threshold of training refer to Chart 4.1, page 147. Optimally you should determine your *own* threshold level from the chart and maintain your heart rate at that level for 30 minutes daily. Refer to page 17 for more information on the cardiovascular threshold of training.

There are some techniques that every jogger should be familiar with before starting a jogging program.

1. *Foot Placement*—The heel of the foot hits the ground first in jogging. Your heel should strike before the rest of the foot (but not vigorously) and then you should rock forward and push off with the ball of your foot. Contrary to some opinion, you should *not* jog on your toes. (A flat foot landing can be all right as long as you push off with the ball of the foot). The toes should point straight ahead. The feet should stay under the knees and should *not* swing out to the sides as you jog.
2. *Length of Stride*—For efficiency you should have a relatively long stride. Your stride should be at least several inches longer than your walking stride. If necessary you may have to "reach" to lengthen your stride. Most older people find it more efficient to run with a shorter stride.

3. *Arm Movement*—While you jog you should work with the arms as well as the legs. The arms should be bent at about 90 degrees and should swing freely and alternately from front to back. The arms should swing in the direction you are moving and not from side to side. Keep the arms and hands relaxed.

4. *Body Position*—While jogging the upper body should be nearly erect. The head and chest should be held up and there should not be a conscious effort to lean forward as is the case in sprinting or fast running.

5. Refer to page 120 for a discussion of some of the common problems experienced by joggers.

Weight Training

Weight training is perhaps the most effective type of training to improve muscular strength. There are as many different weight training exercises as there are different muscles in the body. However, there are a few exercises that require overload of the major muscle groups. These exercises are presented on pages 286-289.

Before beginning a weight training program you should review the guidelines for strength development on Table 6.1 and the Principles of Isotonic Strength on Table 6.2.

Also, prior to beginning a regular weight training program it is important to test yourself to determine the optimal weights to be lifted for each exercise. This is done by trial and error. Begin lifting *too little* weight at first. Determine the maximum amount you can lift for four repetitions of each exercise. Do one set of four repetitions at ½ maximum, the next set at ¾ maximum, and the final set at maximum weight. As you improve, increase the repetitions until you can do eight in each set. Then increase the weight and resume four repetitions.

Advantages and Disadvantages of Weight Training

Advantages	*Disadvantages*
1. Weight training is probably the best method available for developing strength and to a lesser extent muscular endurance.	1. Weight training does little to improve the health-related aspects of physical fitness other than strength and muscular endurance.
2. Weight training can result in significant changes in appearance that are favorable to both men and women.	

A   The Basic Weight Training Exercises

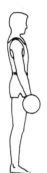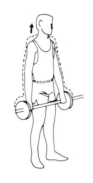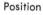

Position   Movement

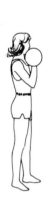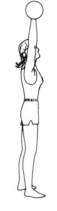

Position   Movement

Shoulder Shrug

Purpose

Strengthen the muscles of the shoulders and arms.

Position

1. Palms toward body.
2. Bar touching thighs.
3. Legs straight.
4. Feet together.

Movement

1. Lift shoulders (try to touch ears).
2. Roll shoulders smoothly backward.
3. Roll shoulders down and forward.
4. Repeat maximum number of times.

Military Press

Purpose

Strengthen the muscles of the shoulders and arms.

Position

1. Palms forward (chest position, front grip).
2. Hands spread (slightly more than shoulder width).
3. Bar touching chest.
4. Feet spread (comfortable distance)
5. Feet flat, legs straight.

Movement

1. Move bar to overhead position (arms straight).
2. Lower to chest position.
3. Repeat.

Half Knee Squats

Purpose

Strengthen the muscles of the thighs and hips.

Position

1. Begin in standing position.
2. Rest bar behind neck on shoulders.
3. Spread hands (comfortable position).
4. Feet at 45° angle.

Movement

1. Squat slowly.
2. Back straight, eyes ahead.
3. Bend knees to 90°, keep knees over feet.
4. Pause, then stand.
5. Repeat.

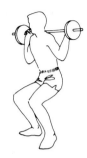

Position   Movement

Curls

Purpose

Strengthen the muscles of the upper front part of the arms.

Position

1. Palms away from body (reverse grip).
2. Arms spread in order not to touch body.
3. Bar touching thighs.
4. Spread feet (comfortable position).

Movement

1. Move bar to chin.
2. Keep body straight.
3. Keep elbows forward of center line of body.
4. Don't allow elbows to touch body.
5. Repeat.

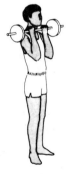

Position   Movement

Elbow Extension Behind Neck

Purpose

Strengthen the muscles of the upper back part of the arms (triceps).

Position

1. Front grip.
2. Hands together at center of bar.
3. Feet spread, body straight.
4. Rest bar behind neck on shoulders.
5. Point elbows upward.

Movement

1. Hold upper arms stationary.
2. Raise weight overhead.
3. Lower bar to neck (reverse movement).
4. Repeat.

Position   Movement

Toe Raises

Purpose

Strengthen muscles of the lower back part of the legs (calf).

Position

1. Front grip.
2. Hands wider than shoulder width apart.
3. Legs straight.
4. Balls of foot resting on 2 inch block with heels on floor.
5. *Variations:*
   (a) Toes together, heels apart.
   (b) Feet apart, toes straight ahead.

Position   Movement

Movement

1. Rise on toes quickly.
2. Hold for one second.
3. Lower heels to floor.
4. Repeat.

Pull to Chin

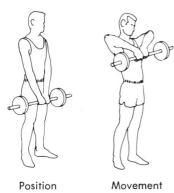

Position   Movement

Purpose

Strengthen muscles of the shoulders and arms.

Position

1. Front grip (loose).
2. Hands together at center of bar.
3. Feet spread, body straight.
4. Head erect, eyes straight ahead.

Movement

1. Pull bar to chin.
2. Keep elbows close to body.
3. Keep elbows well above bar.
4. Lower to extended position.
5. Repeat.

Isometric Exercise

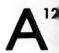

Isometric exercises are intended primarily to develop muscular strength and endurance. Sixteen different exercises for different body parts are presented here. You should select exercises for your program (if you choose isometric exercise) that meet your own personal needs.

Before performing isometric exercises as part of your exercise program you should review the guidelines for strength development on page 33 (Table 6.1) and the Principles of Isometric Exercise on page 34 (Table 6.2).

Advantages and Disadvantages of Isometric Exercises

Advantages

1. Isometrics are good for developing strength and muscular endurance.

2. Isometrics require little equipment and little space.

Disadvantages

1. Isometric exercises do nothing to promote flexibility and cardiovascular fitness. Isometrics should be avoided by those with high blood pressure or heart disease.

2. It may be hard to motivate yourself for maximal contractions.

Isometric Exercises

All of the following exercises should be held for five to eight seconds and should be repeated several times a day.

3. Forearms are parallel to floor.
4. Attempt to pull hands apart with maximum force.

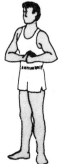

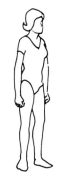

Chest Push

Purpose

Develop muscles of the chest and upper arms.

1. Place palm of right hand in left fist.
2. Keep hands close to chest.
3. Forearms parallel to floor.
4. Push hands together with maximum strength.

Fist Squeeze

Purpose

Develop muscles of the lower arm.

1. Arms extended at side.
2. Clench fists as hard as possible.
3. Repeat.

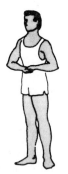

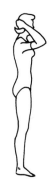

Shoulder Pull

Purpose

Develop muscles of the upper back and arms.

1. Cup hands and interlock fingers.
2. Keep hands close to chest.

Neck Pull

Purpose

Develop muscles of the neck, upper back, and arms.

1. Interlock fingers behind head.
2. Elbows pointing forward.
3. Force head backward.
4. Pull hands forward with maximum strength.

Strengthen Back

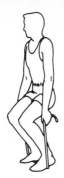

Purpose

Develop muscles of arms, legs, and hips.

1. Loop rope under feet.
2. Stand on rope, feet spread shoulder width.
3. Keep back straight.
4. Bend knees, grasp both ends of rope.
5. Back erect and arms straight, buttocks low.
6. Lift upward with maximum strength.

Overhead Pull

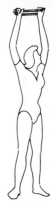

Purpose

Develop muscles of the arms and shoulders.

1. Fold rope in a double loop.
2. Grasp rope overhead, palms outward.
3. Extend arms.
4. Push outward at maximum force.
5. Repeat with palms in.

Curls

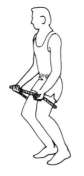

Purpose

Develop muscles of the upper arms.

1. Place rope loop behind thighs while standing in a half squat position.
2. Grasp loop, palms up, shoulder width.
3. Lift upward with maximum strength.
4. For reverse curls, repeat with grip palms down.

Foot Lift

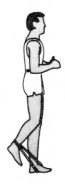

Purpose

Develop muscles of legs.

1. Stand on loop with left foot.
2. Place loop around right ankle.
3. Flex knee until taut.
4. Apply maximum strength upward.
5. Repeat forward, to side, with both feet.

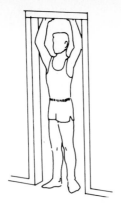

Military Press in Doorway

Purpose

Develop muscles of the arms and shoulders.

1. Stand in doorway.
2. Face straight ahead.
3. Hands shoulders width apart, elbows bent.
4. Tighten leg, hip, and back muscles.
5. Push upward as hard as possible.

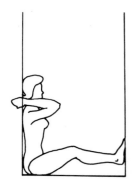

Leg Press in Doorway

Purpose

Develop muscles of the legs.

1. Sit in doorway facing the side of the door frame.
2. Grasp molding behind head.
3. Keep back flat on side of doorway, feet against other side.
4. Push legs with maximum strength.

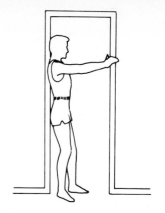

Arm Press in Doorway

Purpose

Develop muscles of the arms.

1. Stand in doorway.
2. Back flat on one side of doorway, hands placed on other side.
3. Push with maximum strength.

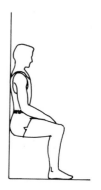

Wall Seat

Purpose

Develop muscles of the leg and hips.

1. Assume half-sit position.
2. Back flat against wall.
3. Knees bent to 90°.
4. Push back against wall with maximum strength.

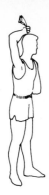

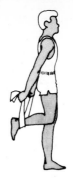

Leg Extension

Purpose

Develop muscles of thigh.

1. Place towel around right ankle.
2. Knee bent at 90° angle.
3. Grasp towel with both hands behind back.
4. Extend leg downward with maximum force.
5. Repeat exercise by changing legs.

Triceps Extension

Purpose

Develop muscles of upper arm.

1. Grasp towel at both ends.
2. Hold left hand at small of back.
3. Right hand over shoulder.
4. Pull towel with maximum force.
5. Repeat exercise by changing position of hands.

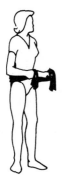

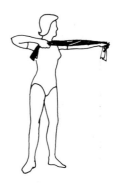

Waist Pull

Purpose

Develop muscles of the abdomen and arms.

1. Grasp ends of towel, palms in.
2. Towel around back of waist.
3. Elbows flexed to right angle.
4. Pull forward on towel with maximum strength while contracting abdomen and flattening back.

Bow Exercise

Purpose

Develop muscles of arms, shoulders and upper back.

1. Take archer's position with bow drawn.
2. Left elbow partially extended.
3. Right hand at chin, right arm parallel to floor.
4. Grasp towel and pull arms away from each other.
5. Exchange positions of hands and repeat.

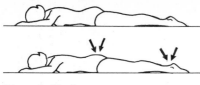

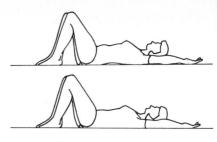

Gluteal Pinch

Purpose

Develop muscles of the buttocks.

1. Lie prone, heels apart and big toes touching.
2. Pinch the buttocks together; hold several seconds.
3. Slowly relax.
4. Repeat several times.

Pelvic Tilt

Purpose

Develop muscles of the abdomen and buttocks.

1. Assume a supine position with the knees bent and slightly apart.
2. Press the spine down on the floor and hold for five seconds.
3. Keep tightened abdominals and gluteals.

A¹³   Isotonic Exercises for Muscular Endurance and Mild Strengthening

The exercises suggested here should be performed as described until the person is able to increase the repetitions to approximately twenty-five or more for some exercises; then additional weight should be added.

Advantages and Disadvantages of Isotonic Exercises for People with Limited Strength

Advantages	*Disadvantages*
1. Suitable for persons of a wide range of strength levels.	1. These exercises will not increase cardiovascular fitness and have only limited ability to increase strength.
2. Suitable for figure or physique control and postural correction.	
3. Designed for muscular endurance and mild strengthening.	

The Isotonic Exercises

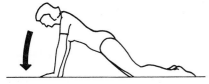

Bent Knee Let-downs

For those who cannot do bent knee push-ups.

Purpose

Develop muscles of the arms, shoulders, and chest.

Let-downs

Assume a bent knee push-up position and slowly lower the body to the floor, keeping the body line straight; return to the starting position in any manner.

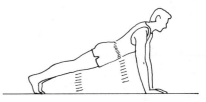

Full-length Push-ups

Purpose

Develop muscles of arms and chest.

Full-length Push-ups

Take front-leaning rest position, arms straight. Lower chest to floor. Press to beginning position in same manner. Repeat exercise as many times as possible up to thirty-five.

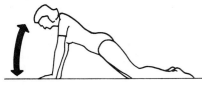

Bent Knee Push-ups

For those who cannot do full-length push-up.

Purpose

Develop muscles of the arms, shoulders, and chest.

Push-ups

Assume the push-up position (as in No. 1). Lower the body until the chest touches the floor; return to the starting position keeping the body straight.

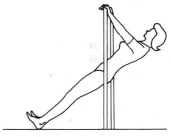

Modified Pull-ups

Purpose

Develop muscles of the arms, shoulders, and chest.

Pull-ups

Hang (palms forward and shoulder width apart) from a low bar (may be placed across two chairs), heels on floor, with the body straight from feet to head; pull up, keeping the body straight, and touch the chest to the bar, then lower to the starting position. (Stronger persons may hang from a bar vertically and pull up).

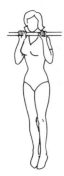

Pull Ups (Chinning)

Purpose

Develop muscles of arms and shoulders.

Pull Ups (Chinning)

Grasp bar, palms forward, arms and body straight. Lift chin to bar. Press to beginning position in same manner. Repeat exercise as many times as possible up to thirty-five.

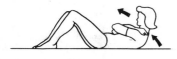

Bent Knee Sit-ups

Purpose

Develop the upper abdominal muscles and correct ptosis.

Sit-ups

Assume a hook-lying position with the arms crossed and the hands on the shoulders; roll up, making the elbows touch the knees, then roll down to the starting position.

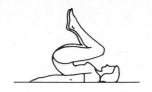

Reverse Sit-ups

Purpose

Develop the lower abdominal muscles and correct abdominal ptosis.

Reverse Sit-ups

Lie on the floor, bend the knees, place the feet flat on the floor, and place arms at sides; lift the knees to the chest raising the hips off the floor; return to the starting position.

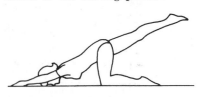

Leg Extension Exercise

Purpose

Develop muscles of the hips.

Leg Extension

Assume a knee-chest position, hands on floor with arms extended as far as possible; extend right leg upward in line with trunk; then lower. Continue repetitions, repeat with other leg.

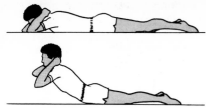

Prone Back Lift

Purpose

Develop muscles of the upper back. Correct kyphosis and round shoulders.

Prone Back Lift

Lie prone (face down) with hands clasped behind the neck. Pull the shoulder blades together, raising the elbows off the floor; slowly raise the head and chest off the floor by arching the upper back; return to the starting position; repeat. Caution: Do not arch the lower back; lift only until the sternum (breast bone) clears the floor.

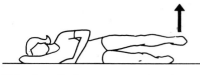

Side Leg Raises

Purpose

Develop muscles on outside of thighs.

Side Leg Raise

Lie on the side and raise the top leg toward the ceiling, then return. Do all repetitions with each leg.

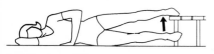

Lower Leg Lift

Purpose

Develop muscles on the inside of the thighs.

Lower Leg Lift

Lie on the side with the upper leg (foot) supported on a bench; raise the lower leg toward the ceiling; repeat on opposite side.

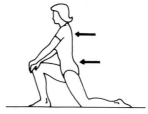

Stride Squat

Purpose

Develop muscles of the legs and hips.

Stride Squat

Stand tall, feet together. Take a long step forward with the left foot touching the right knee to the floor. Return to the starting position and step out with the other foot. Repeat, alternating left and right.

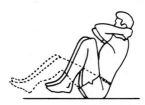

Sitting Tucks or "V Sit"

Purpose

Develop muscles of abdomen and legs.

Sitting Tucks or "V Sit"

Sit on the floor so that the back and feet are off the floor. Interlock fingers behind the head. Alternately draw the legs into the chest and extend the feet away from the body. Keep feet and back off the floor. Repeat as many times as possible up to thirty-five.

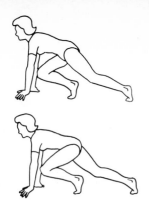

Stationary Leg Change

Purpose

Develop muscles of the legs and hips.

Stationary Leg Change

Crouch on the floor with weight on hands, left leg bent under the chest, right leg extended behind. Alternate legs; bring right leg up while left leg goes back. Repeat as many times as possible up to fifty.

A¹⁴   Flexibility Exercises

Before you use flexibility exercises in your regular program of exercise you should review the guidelines for flexibility development on page 43 (Table 7.2) and the table comparing the advantages of passive and ballistic flexibility exercises on page 42 (Table 7.1).

Specific instructions for performing each exercise are provided opposite each exercise illustration.

Advantages and Disadvantages of a Flexibility Exercise Program

Advantages	*Disadvantages*
1. Flexibility exercises can serve as "limbering up" exercises in addition to developing flexibility.	1. Flexibility exercises do not promote all health-related fitness aspects.
2. Flexibility exercises can compliment strength and muscular endurance exercises and keep muscles from becoming too short or "musclebound."	

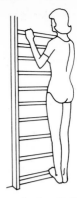

1. To Stretch the Calf Muscles and Achilles Tendons. Stand with the toes on a thick book or lower rung of a stall bar; hold on to a support with hands; lower heels toward floor as far as possible; hold several seconds. Repeat several times. If a ballistic stretch is desired, bounce gently.

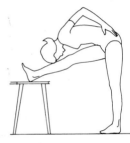

2. To Stretch Lower Back and Hamstring Muscles. Stand with one foot on a bench; keeping the leg straight, bend the trunk forward, trying to touch the head to the knee; hold for a few seconds; return to starting position and repeat with opposite leg. As flexibility improves the arms can be used to pull the chest toward the legs. Useful in relief of backache and correction of lordosis. If a ballistic stretch is desired, bounce gently.

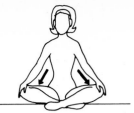

3. To Stretch Muscles on Inside of Thighs. Sit with the knees apart and the legs crossed at the ankles. Place the hands on the inside of the knees and push toward the floor. Hold for several seconds and repeat. Useful for pregnant women or anyone whose thighs tend to rotate inward causing knock-knees and foot pronation.

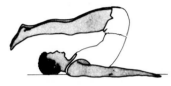

4. To Stretch the Lower Back. Lie supine, arms at side, draw bent knees to chest, then straighten legs so they are over the head and trunk, parallel to floor (do not allow buttocks to go beyond head); hold several seconds; return to starting position by bringing bent knees back to chest. Repeat several times. Avoid getting the weight over the neck and avoid straight-leg lowering. Useful for backache and lordosis.

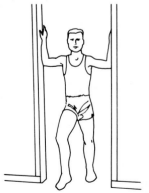

5. Pectoral Stretch. Stand erect in doorway with arms raised shoulder height, elbows bent and hands grasping doorjambs; step forward with either foot, forcing chest forward; repeat several times. Useful for round shoulders, kyphosis, and sunken chest.

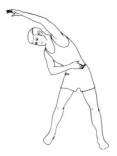

6. Lateral Trunk Flexibility. Stand with feet shoulders width apart, hands on hips. Stretch left arm over head to right. Bend to right at waist reaching as far to right as possible with left arm. Repeat to left side with right arm reaching over head to left. Repeat several times.

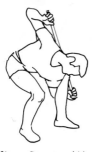

7. Flexibility Stunt. (A) Grasp a broomstick, or wand, with hands palm down about shoulder's width apart; (B) Reach the end of broomstick and the left hand between the legs; (C) Step with left leg around the outside of the arm and between the stick and the body; (D) Slide the stick over the left knee, left hip, and back; and (E) Step the right foot over the stick and stand holding the stick in front of body, palms up.

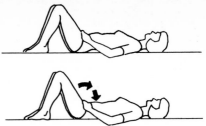

8. Mosher Exercise — For Relief of Dysmenorrhea. In a supine position with the knees bent and feet on the floor, suck in the abdomen and tip the pelvis backward. Try to press the low back flat against the floor. Hold for six seconds, then try to "blow up" abdomen (balloon), pushing it out until it stretches. Relax and repeat.

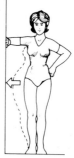

9. Billig's Exercise — For Dysmenorrhea (painful menstruation). Menstrual cramps are a problem experienced by many women. This exercise, if done regularly, can help relieve menstrual pain. This exercise can be done before exercise or it can be done as a part of your regular exercise program. The exercise is for women, but men may choose to learn the exercise so that they may pass it on to women who may benefit from it.

Stand with side to a wall and place the elbow and forearm against the wall at shoulder height. *Tilt the pelvis backward tightening the gluteal and abdominal muscles.* Place opposite hand on hip and push the hips toward the wall. Push forward and sideward (45°) with the hips. *Do not twist the hips.* A stretch should be felt in the abdominal region. Hold this position for several seconds. Keep knees straight and the chest high. Repeat several times as necessary.

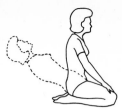

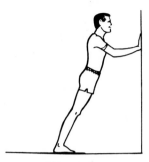

10. **Sore calf muscles** are another problem common to people who participate in regular exercise. Passive stretching of the calf muscles during a warm-up can help relieve the soreness of these muscles. Some suggest that this exercise can be of benefit if performed after exercise as well as during the warm-up; also good conditioning for snow skiing.

Face the wall with feet together three to four feet from the wall. Keeping the body straight lean forward and support the upper body on the wall. Keep the heels on the floor. Hold for six to twelve seconds, stretching the calf muscles and Achilles tendon.

11. **Exercises for Leg Soreness (Shin Splints).** "Shin splints" are a common source of muscle pain that results from exercise, particularly exercise that involves bouncing on the legs, such as in basketball or even jogging on a hard surface. Regular passive stretching can help reduce "shin splint" soreness. This exercise may be performed before your regular exercise program as a warm-up. Some suggest that it may be done after exercise as a prevention against future soreness. NOTE: If pain persists, is severe, or other evidence of muscle injury exists, discontinue this exercise until you get a medical diagnosis of the exact nature of your problem.

Kneel with the front of the lower leg in contact with the floor. The toes should be pointed backward with the top of the foot in contact with the floor. Gently lean the upper body back thus stretching the "shin" muscles (also good to increase strength of abdominals and hip flexors on the return movement).

References

1. Allsop, G. "Potential Hazards of Abdominal Exercises." *Journal of Health, Physical Education and Recreation* 89:January, 1971.
2. "All the News That's Fit." *Fitness for Living* 15:July-August, 1971.
3. American Alliance for Health, Physical Education and Recreation. *Nutrition for Athletes.* Washington, D. C., 1971.
4. American Medical Association. *Merchants of Menace.* Chicago: AMA, 1966.
5. Anderson, C. L. *Community Health.* St. Louis: The C. V. Mosby Co., 1969, p. 124.
6. Appleton, S. F., et al. "Weight Reduction Industry." Unpublished study. University of California, Berkeley, 1971.
7. Arnheim, D. D.; Auxter, D.; and Crowe, W. D. *Principles and Methods of Adapted Physical Education.* 3rd ed. St. Louis: C. V. Mosby Co., 1977.
8. Astrand, P. O. "Diet and Athletic Performance." *Nutrition Today* 3:9, 1968.
9. Astrand, P. O. and Rodahl, K. *Textbook of Work Physiology.* New York: McGraw-Hill, 1970.
10. Balke, B. "The Effects of Physical Exercise on Metabolic Potential, A Crucial Measure of Physical Fitness." *Exercises and Fitness.* Chicago: Athletic Institute, 1960.
11. Barber, T. X., et al., ed. *Biofeedback and Self-Control.* Chicago: Aldine-Atherton, 1971.
12. Barnard, R. J. "The Heart Needs a Warm-up Time." *The Physician and Sports Medicine* 4:40, 1976.
13. Bassler, T. J. "Marathon Running and Immunity to Heart Disease." *The Physician and Sports Medicine* 3:77, 1975.
14. Benson, H. *The Relaxation Response.* New York: William Morrow and Company, Inc., 1975.
15. Berger, R. A. "Effect of Varied Weight Training Programs on Strength." *Research Quarterly* 33:121, 1966.
16. ———. "Effects of Dynamic and Static Training on Vertical Jump Ability." *Research Quarterly* 34:419, 1963.
17. ———. "Relationship Between Dynamic Strength and Dynamic Endurance." *Research Quarterly* 41:115, 1970.
18. Bergstrom, J. and Hultman, E. "Nutrition for Maximal Sports Performance." *Journal of the American Medical Association* 221:992, August 28, 1972.
19. Billig, H. E., and Loewendall, E. *Mobilization of the Human Body.* Stanford, Cal.: Stanford University Press, 1949.
20. Blievernicht, J. "Accuracy in the Tennis Forehand Drive: Cinematographic Analysis." *Research Quarterly* 39:776, October, 1968.
21. Bogert, L. J., et al. *Nutrition and Physical Fitness,* 9th ed. Philadelphia: W. B. Saunders Company, 1973.

22. Boye, J. "Exercise and Blood Cholesterol." *Physical Fitness Research Digest* 3:6, July, 1972.

23. Boyer, J. L. "Effects of Chronic Exercise on Cardiovascular Function." *Physical Fitness Research Digest* 2:1, 1972.

24. ———. "Mechanisms by Which Physical Activity May Reduce the Occurrence or Severity of Coronary Heart Disease." *Physical Fitness Research Digest* 2:1, October, 1972.

25. ——— and Kash, F. W. "Exercise Therapy in Hypertensive Men." *Journal of the American Medical Association* 10:1668, March, 1970.

26. Bridell, G. E. "A Comparison of Selected Static and Dynamic Stretching Exercises on the Flexibility of the Hip Joint." *Completed Research in Health, Physical Education and Recreation* 12:209, 1970.

27. Broer, R. *Efficiency of Human Movement*, 3rd ed. Philadelphia: W. B. Saunders Co., 1973.

28. Brown, L. H. and Wilmore, J. H. "The Effects of Maximal Resistance Training on the Strength and Body Composition of Women Athletes." *Medicine and Science in Sports* 6:174, 1974.

29. Brumfield, M. D. "A Comparison of the Relationship of Shoulder Flexibility and Other Selected Factors to Throwing Performances by College Women." *Completed Research in Health, Physical Education and Recreation* 12:218, 1970.

30. Bruner, D. and Manelis, G. "Myocardial Infarction Among Members of Communal Settlements in Israel." *Lancet* 2:1049, 1960.

31. Bunn, J. *Scientific Principles of Coaching*. Englewood Cliffs, New Jersey: Prentice-Hall, Inc., 1972.

32. Bunnell, R. H., et al. "Effect of Feeding Polyunsaturated Fatty Acids with a Low Vitamin E Diet on Blood Levels of Tocopherol in Men Performing Hard Physical Labor." *American Journal of Clincal Nutrition* 28:706, July, 1975.

33. Burt, J. J.; Blyth, C. S.; and Rierson, H. A. "Effects of Exercise on the Coagulation—Fibrinolysis Equilibrium." *Journal of Sports Medicine and Physical Fitness* 4:213, 1964.

34. Burt, J. J. and Jackson, R. "The Effects of Physical Exercise on the Coronary Collateral Circulation of Dogs." *Journal of Sports Medicine and Physical Fitness* 5:203, 1965.

35. Bushey, S. R. "Relationship of Modern Dance Performance to Agility, Balance, Flexibility, Power and Strength." *Research Quarterly* 37:313, 1966.

36. Butler, R. N. "Psychological Importance of Physical Fitness." *Testimony on Physical Fitness for Older Persons*. Washington, D. C.: National Association for Human Development, 1975.

37. Carlson, R. B. "Relative Isometric Endurance and Different Levels of Athletic Achievement." *Research Quarterly* 40:475, 1969.

38. ——— and McCraw, L. W. "Isometric Strength and Relative Isometric Endurance." *Research Quarterly* 42:244, 1971.

39. Carlsoo, S. *How Man Moves*. London: Heinemann, 1972.

40. Carr, R. *The Yoga Way to Release Tension*. New York: Coward, McCann & Geoghegan, Inc., 1974.

41. Child, I. L. and Whiting, J. W. "Determinants of Level of Aspiration: Evidence of Everyday Life." *Journal of Abnormal Social Psychology* 44: 303, 1949.

42. Clarke, D. H. "Adaptations in Strength and Muscular Endurance Re-

sulting from Exercise," in *Exercise and Sport Sciences Reviews*. Edited by Jack H. Wilmore. New York: Academic Press, 1973, pp. 74-102.

43. ——— and Henry, F. M. "Neuromuscular Specificity and Increased Speed from Strength Development." *Research Quarterly* 32:315, 1961.

44. ——— and Stull, G. A. "Endurance Training as a Determinant of Strength and Fatigability." *Research Quarterly* 41:19, 1970.

45. Clarke, H. H., ed. "Development of Muscular Strength and Endurance." *Physical Fitness Research Digest* 4:1, 1974.

46. ———, ed. "Diet and Exercise in Relation to Peripheral Vascular Disease." *Physical Fitness Research Digest* 6:11, 1976.

47. ———, ed. "Exercise and Fat Reduction." *Physical Fitness Research Digest* 5:1, 1975.

48. ———, ed. "Strength Development and Motor Sports Improvement." *Physical Fitness Research Digest* 4:1, October, 1974.

49. ———, ed. "Toward a Better Understanding of Muscular Strength." *Physical Fitness Research Digest* 3:1, January, 1973.

50. Compton, D., et al. "Weight Lifter's Blackout." *Lancet*, 1234, December, 1973.

51. Conrad, C. C. "Physical Fitness for the Elderly." *Testimony on Physical Fitness for Older Persons*. Washington, D. C.: National Association for Human Development, 1975.

52. ———. "How Different Sports Rate in Promoting Physical Fitness." *Medical Times* 104:65, May, 1976.

53. Consolazio, C. F. "Physical Activity and Performance of the Adolescent," in McKigney, J. I., et al. *Nutrient Requirements in Adolescence*. Cambridge, Mass: MIT Press, 1976, pp. 203-21.

54. Consolazio, C. F., et al. "Protein Metabolism During Intensive Physical Training in the Young Adult." *American Journal of Clinical Nutrition* 28:29, January, 1975.

55. Cooper, D. "Drugs and the Athlete." *Journal of the American Medical Association* 221:1107, August 28, 1972.

56. Cooper, K. H. "A Means of Assessing Maximal Oxygen Uptake." *Journal of the American Medical Association* 203-201, January, 1968.

57. ——— and Cooper, M. *Aerobics for Women*. New York: M. Evans & Co., Inc., 1972.

58. ———. *The New Aerobics*. New York: M. Evans and Company, Inc. 1970.

59. Corbin, C. B. "Effects of Mental Practice and Skill Development After Controlled Practice." *Research Quarterly* 38:534, 1967.

60. ———. "The Effects of Covert Rehearsal on the Development of a Complex Motor Skill." *Journal of General Psychology* 76:143, 1967.

61. ——— and Pletcher, P. "Diet and Physical Activity Patterns of Obese and Nonobese Elementary School Children." *Research Quarterly* 39:922, 1968

62. ———. *Becoming Physically Educated in the Elementary School*, 2d edition. Philadelphia: Lea & Febiger, 1976.

63. ———. "Overload." *Encyclopedia of Sport Sciences and Medicine*. New York: Macmillan, 1971.

64. ———. "A Study of Spectator Attitudes About Sportsmanship." *Texas Association of Health, Physical Education and Recreation Journal* 40:6, 1971.

65. ———. *A Textbook of Motor Development*. Dubuque, Iowa: Wm. C. Brown Co. Publishers, 1973.

66. ———. "Mental Practice." A chapter in *Ergogenic Aids and Muscular Per-*

formance. Morgan, W. P., ed. New York: Academic Press, 1972, pp. 94-116.

67. Costill, D. L., et al. "Water and Electrolyte Replacement During Repeated Days of Work in the Heat." *Aviation Space Environmental Medicine* 46: 795, June, 1975.

68. Cratty, B. J. *Psychology and Physical Activity.* Englewood Cliffs, N. J.: Prentice-Hall, 1968.

69. ———. *Social Dimensions of Physical Activity.* Englewood Cliffs, N. J.: Prentice-Hall, 1967.

70. Creus, J. and Aldinger, E. E. "Effects of Chronic Exercise on Myocardial Function." *American Heart Journal* 74:537, 1967.

71. Cundiff, D. E. *Fundamentals of Functional Fitness.* Dubuque, Iowa: Kendall/Hunt, 1974.

72. Darda, G. *A Method of Determining the Relative Contributions of the Diver and Springboard to the Vertical Ascent of the Forward Three and One-Half Somersaults Tuck.* Doctoral dissertation, University of Wisconsin, 1972.

73. Davies, G. B. "Exercises: Good, Bad, and Indifferent." *Journal of Health, Physical Education and Recreation* 24:14, January, 1953.

74. Dawber, T. R. "Risk Factors in Young Adults: The Lessons from Epidemiologic Studies of Cardiovascular Disease—Framingham, Tecumseh, and Evans County." *Journal of the American College Health Association* 22:84, 1973.

75. "Deep Bending Exercises May Be the Lower Back's Last Straw." *Medical World News* 96, June 2, 1967.

76. deVries, H. A. "Electromyographic Observations of the Effects of Static Stretching Upon Muscular Distress." *Research Quarterly* 32:468, 1961.

77. ———. "Evaluation of Static Stretching Procedures for Improvement of Flexibility." *Research Quarterly* 33:222, 1962.

78. ———. *Physiology of Exercise.* Dubuque, Iowa: Wm. C. Brown Co. Publishers, 1974.

79. ———. "Prevention of Muscular Distress After Exercise." *Research Quarterly* 32:177, 1961.

80. ———. "What Research Tells Us Regarding the Contribution of Exercise to the Health of Older People." *Testimony on the Physical Fitness of Older People.* Washington, D. C.: National Association for Human Development, 3-7, 1975.

81. Dodge, D. L. and Martin, W. T. *Social Stress and Chronic Illness.* Notre Dame, Ind.: University of Notre Dame Press, 1970.

82. Droescher, J. *A Mechanical Analysis of the Front Somersault Between the Uneven Parallel Bars.* Doctoral dissertation, Springfield College, 1973.

83. Dvorak, R. *A Kinematic Comparison Between the Bent and Straight Arm Giant Swing on the Still Rings Using Cinematographical Analysis.* Doctoral dissertation, University of New Mexico, 1973.

84. Ecker, T. "Angle of Release in Shot Putting." *Athletic Journal* 50:52, February, 1970.

85. ———. "The Sprinter's Acceleration and Forward Lean." *Athletic Journal* 50:28, April, 1970.

86. ———. "The 20-Foot Vault is Coming." *Athletic Journal* 51:22, February, 1971.

87. Eckstein, R. "Effect of Exercise and Coronary Artery Narrowing on Coronary Collateral Circulation." *Circulation Research* 5:230, 1957.

88. Ellis, M. J. *Why People Play.* Englewood Cliffs, N. J.: Prentice-Hall, 1973.

89. Elrich, H. "Exercise and the Aging Process." *Testimony on Physical Fitness for Older Persons.* Washington, D. C.: National Association for Human Development, 1975.

90. *Facts on the Killing and Crippling Diseases in the United States Today.* New York: The National Health Education Committee, Inc., 1964.

91. Fahrni, W. H. *Backache Relieved Through New Concepts of Posture.* Springfield, Ill.: Charles C Thomas, Publisher, 1966.

92. Fait, H. F. *Special Physical Education: Adapted, Corrective, Developmental,* 3d ed. Philadelphia: W. B. Saunders Co., 1972.

93. Farfan, H. F. *Mechanical Disorders of the Low Back.* Philadelphia: Lea & Febiger, 1973.

94. Faria, I. E. "Cardiovascular Response to Exercise as Influenced by Training of Various Intensities." *Research Quarterly* 41:44, 1970.

95. Fast, J. *Body Language.* New York: Pocket Books, 1971.

96. *Federal Trade Commission News,* July 23, 1970, Washington, D. C.

97. Feffer, H. L. "All About Backaches—Latest Advice from a Specialist." *U.S. News and World Report* 71:74, September 20, 1971.

98. Finneson, B. E. *Low Back Pain.* Philadelphia: J. B. Lippincott Co., 1973.

99. Fisher, A. C. *Psychology of Sport.* Palo Alto, Cal.: Mayfield, 1976.

100. Flint, M. M. "Effect of Increasing Back and Abdominal Muscle Strength on Low Back Pain." *Research Quarterly* 29:160, 1958.

101. ———. "Selecting Exercises." *Journal of Health, Physical Education and Recreation* 35:19, February, 1964.

102. Fox, S. M.; Naughton, J. P.; and Skinner, J. S. "Physical Activity in Prevention of Coronary Heart Disease." *Annals of Clinical Research* 3:404, 1971.

103. Freed, D. L. J., et al. "Anabolic Steroids in Athletics: Crossover Double-blind Trial on Weightlifters." *British Medical Journal* 2:471, May, 1975.

104. Fried, J. J. "Biofeedback: Teaching Your Body to Heal Itself." *Family Health,* February, 1974, and *Reader's Digest* May, 1974, p. 110.

105. Friedman, L. W. and Galton, L. *Freedom from Backaches.* New York: Simon & Schuster, 1973.

106. Gench, B. E. "Cardiovascular Adaptations for College Women to Training at Predetermined Individualized Heart Rate Levels for Varied Durations." *The Foil* 56, 1975.

107. Gerber, E. W., et al. *The American Woman in Sport.* Reading, Mass.: Addison-Wesley, 1974.

108. Glass, D. C. and Singer, J. E. *Urban Stress: Experiments on Noise and Social Stressors.* New York: Academic Press, 1972.

109. Goldberg, A. L., et al. "Mechanism of Work-Induced Hypertrophy of Skeletal Muscle." *Medicine and Science in Sports* 7:248, 1975.

110. Golding, L. A. "Cholesterol and Exercise, A Ten Year Study." *Journal of Physical Education* 69:106, March-April, 1972.

111. Grandjean, E. *Fitting the Task to the Man.* London: Taylor and Francis, Ltd., 1969.

112. Gunderson, E.K.E. and Rahe, R. H., ed. *Life Stress and Illness.* Springfield, Ill.: Charles C Thomas, Publisher, 1974.

113. Haley, P. R., "A Comparative Analysis of Selected Motor Fitness Test Performance of Elementary School Boys. *Dissertation Abstracts International* 32:5018A, 1972.

114. Hannum, S. "Spring Has Sprung." *San Diego State University Adult Fitness Program Newsletter,* April, 1976.

115. Harger, B. S. et al. "The Caloric Cost of Running—Its Impact on Weight Reduction," *Journal of The American Medical Association* 228:483, April 22, 1974.

116. Harris, M. L. "A Factor Analysis of Flexibility." *Research Quarterly* 40:62, 1969.

117. Harvey, V. P. and Scott, G. D. "Reliability of a Measure of Forward Flexibility and Its Relationship to Physical Dimensions of College Women." *Research Quarterly* 38:28, 1967.

118. Haslam, R. W. and Stull, G. A. "Duration and Frequency of Training as Determinants of Coronary Tree Capacity of Rats." *Research Quarterly* 45:178, 1974.

119. Hassard, G. H. and Redd, C. L. *Elongation Treatment of Low Back Pain.* Springfield, Ill.: Charles C Thomas, Publisher, 1959.

120. Hay, J. *An Investigation of Mechanical Efficiency in Two Styles of High Jumping.* Doctoral dissertation, University of Iowa, 1967.

121. ———. *Biomechanics of Sports Techniques.* Englewood Cliffs, N. J.: Prentice-Hall, Inc., 1973.

122. Hay, G. "The Hay Technique—Ultimate In High Jump Style." *Athletic Journal* 53:46, March, 1973.

123. Hernlund, V. and Steinhaus, A. H. "Do Mechanical Vibrators Take Off or Redistribute Fat?" *Journal of the Association of Physical and Mental Rehabilitation* 11:3:96, 1957.

124. Hinson, M. and Rosenswieg, J. "Comparing the Three Best Ways of Developing Strength." *Scholastic Coach* 41:34, 1972.

125. Hodgson, J. D. "Leisure and the American Worker." *Journal of Health, Physical Education and Recreation* 43:38, 1972.

126. Hollozy, J. O. and Skinner, J. "Effects of Six Months of Endurance Exercise on Serum Lipids of Middle Age Men." *American Journal of Cardiology* 14:753, 1964.

127. Hood, W. "A More Scientific Approach to Shot Putting." *Athletic Journal* 51:59, April, 1971.

128. Holt, L. E., et al. "Comparative Study of Three Stretching Techniques." *Perceptual and Motor Skills* 31:611, 1970.

129. Howland, I. S. *Body Alignment in Fundamental Motor Skills.* New York: Exposition Press, 1953.

130. Hoyman, H. S. "An Ecological View of Health and Health Education," in *Science and Theory of Health: A Book of Readings.* Jones, H. L., Schult, M. B. and Shelton, A. L., eds. Dubuque, Iowa: Wm. C. Brown Company Publishers, 1966, p. 3.

131. Hunt, Valerie. "Movement Behavior: A Model for Action." *Quest* 2:26, 1964.

132. "Ideas on Bedding and Backaches." *Forecast for Home Economics* 19:44, May, 1974.

133. Ishmael, W. K. and Shorbe, H. B. *Care of the Back.* Philadelphia: J. B. Lippincott Co., 1953.

134. Jackson, A. S. and Frankiewicz, R. J. "Factorial Expressions of Muscular Strength." *Research Quarterly* 46:206, May, 1975.

135. Jackson, A. S., et al. "Revision of the AAHPER Youth Fitness Test." A position paper presented to the AAHPER national convention, Milwaukee, Wisc., March, 1976.

136. Jackson, D. W. and Wiltse, L. L. "Low Back Pain in Young Athletes." *The Physician and Sports Medicine* 2:53, 1974.

137. Jacobson, E. *Anxiety and Tension Control.* Philadelphia: J. B. Lippincott Company, 1964.

138. ———. *Modern Treatment of Tense Patients.* Springfield, Ill.: Charles C Thomas, Publisher, 1970.

139. Jensen, R. and Schultz, W. *Applied Kinesiology.* New York: McGraw-Hill, 1970.

140. Johnson, M. L., et al. "Relative Importance of Inactivity and Overeating in Energy Balance of Obese High School Girls." *American Journal of Clinical Nutrition* 4:37, 1956.

141. ———. "The Prevalence and Incidence of Obesity in a Cross Section of Elementary and Secondary School Children." *American Journal of Clinical Nutrition* 4:231, 1956.

142. Johnson, P. B., et al. *Physical Education: A Problem-solving Approach to Health and Fitness.* New York: Holt, Rinehart and Winston, 1966.

143. Jones, L. *The Postural Complex.* Springfield, Ill.: Charles C Thomas, Publisher, 1955.

144. Kannel, W. B. "Habitual Level of Physical Activity and Risk of Coronary Heart Disease." *Canadian Medical Association Journal* 96:811, 1967.

145. Kannel, W. B., et al. "The Framingham Study." *American Journal of Internal Medicine* 74:1, 1971.

146. ———.; Sorlie, P.; and McNamara, P. "The Relation of Physical Activity to Risk of Coronary Heart Disease: The Framingham Study." In *Coronary Heart Disease and Physical Fitness,* edited by O. A. Larsen and R. O. Malmborg. Baltimore: University Park Press, 1971.

147. Karpovich, P. V. "Ergogenic Aids in Athletics." In *Exercise and Fitness,* edited by T. Cureton. Chicago: Athletic Institute, 1966, pp. 82-90.

148. ———. *Physiology of Muscular Activity,* 5th ed. Philadelphia: W. B. Saunders Co., 1959.

149. Karvonen, M. J. "Effects of Vigorous Exercise on the Heart." In *Work and the Heart,* edited by F. F. Rosenbaum and E. L. Belknap. New York: Paul B. Hoebner, 1959.

150. Kasch, F. W. "The Effects of Exercise on the Aging Process." *The Physician and Sports Medicine* 4:65, 1976.

151. ——— and Boyer, J. L. *Adult Fitness: Principles and Practices.* Palo Alto, Cal.: Mayfield, 1968.

152. Kavanaugh, T. "Postcoronary Joggers Need Precise Guidelines." *The Physician and Sports Medicine* 4:63, 1976.

153. Kavanagh, T., et al. "Intensive Exercise in Coronary Rehabilitation." *Medicine and Science in Sports* 5:34, 1973.

154. Kelly, E. D. *Adapted and Corrective Physical Education,* 4th ed. New York: Ronald Press Company, 1965.

155. Kennedy, J. F. "The Soft American." *Sports Illustrated* 13:15, December, 1960.

156. Kenyon, G. S. "Six Scales for Assisting Attitudes Toward Physical Activity." *Research Quarterly* 39:566, 1968.

157. ———. "Values Held for Physical Activity by Selected Urban Secondary School Students in Canada, Australia, England and the United States." A paper available from ERIC Reproduction Services, ED 019 709.

158. Keys, A. and Buzina, R. "Blood Coagulability Effects of Meals and Differences Between Population." *Circulation* 14:479, 1956.

159. Klein, K. K. *The Knees: Growth, Development and Activity Influence.* Greeley, Colo.: All American Publications, 1967.

160. ———. *The Knee in Sports,* 2d ed. Austin, Texas: Pemberton Press, 1971.

161. Klump, F. from "Overcoming Overprotection of the Elderly." *The Physician and Sports Medicine* 4:107, 1976.

162. Klumpp, T. G. "Physical Activities and Older Americans." *Testimony on Physical Fitness for Older Persons.* Washington, D. C.: National Association for Human Development, 1975.

163. Knittle, J. L. and Hirsch, J. "Effect of Early Nutrition and the Development of Rat Epididymal Fat Pads: Cellulasity and Metabolism." *The Journal of Clinical Investigation* 47:2091, 1968.

164. Kournakis, P. "Pharmacological Conditioning for Sporting Events." *American Journal of Pharmacy* 144:151, September-October, 1972.

165. Kraus, H. *Backache, Stress, and Tension.* New York: Simon & Schuster, 1965.

166. ———. "Ecology and Backache." *Journal of Physical Education* 69:111, March, 1972.

167. ——— and Raab, W. *Hypokinetic Disease.* Springfield: Charles C Thomas, Publisher, 1961.

168. Kraus, H. and Weber, S. "Passive and Active Stretching of Muscles." *The Physical Therapy Review* 29:407, September, 1949.

169. Krusen, F. H., et al. *Handbook of Physical Medicine and Rehabilitation,* 2d ed. Philadelphia: W. B. Saunders Company, 1971.

170. Kugelmass, J. A. "How to Keep from Getting Tired." *Capper's Farmer* May, 1959.

171. Kuntzleman, C. "Dangerous Exercise: Which, When, Why." *Fitness for Living* January-February, 1971.

172. Lamb, L. E. "Blood Pressure." *The Health Letter* 1:104, 1973.

173. ———. "Exercise, Heart and Circulation—Part 1." *The Health Letter* 1:1, 1973.

174. ———. "Playboy's Jogging Prank." *The Health Letter* 7:1, 1976.

175. ———. "Staying Youthful and Fit." *Testimony on Physical Fitness for Older Persons.* Washington, D. C.: National Association for Human Development, 1975.

176. Lawrence, J. D., et al. "Effects of Alpha-tocopherol Acetate on the Swimming Endurance of Training Swimmers." *American Journal of Clinical Nutrition* 28:205, March, 1975.

177. Lawther, J. D. *The Learning of Physical Skills.* Englewood Cliffs, N. J.: Prentice-Hall, 2d ed., 1977.

178. ———. *Sport Psychology.* Englewood Cliffs, N. J.: Prentice-Hall, 1972, p. 28.

179. Lewis, S. and Gutin, B. "Nutrition and Endurance." *American Journal of Clinical Nutrition* 26:1011, September, 1973.

180. Lindsey, R., et al. "A Survey and Critical Analysis of Practices Found in Selected Commercial Reducing Salons." Unpublished paper, Oklahoma State University, Stillwater, Okla., 1971.

181. ———. *Body Mechanics,* 3rd ed. Dubuque, Iowa: Wm. C. Brown Company Publishers, 1973.

182. ———. "Figure Wrapping: Can You Believe It?" *Fitness for Living* p. 54, March-April, 1972.

183. Little, C. "The Athlete's Neurosis—A Deprivation Crisis." *Acta Psychiatrica Scandinavica* 45:187, 1969.

184. Logan, G. A. and Egstrom, G. H. "Effects of Slow and Fast Stretching on the Sacrofemoral Angle." *Journal of the Association of Physical and Mental Rehabilitation* 15:85, May-June, 1961.

185. Lowman, C. L. "Faulty Posture in Relation to Performance." *Journal of Health, Physical Education and Recreation* 29:14, April, 1958.

186. McDonald, G. A. and Fullerton, H. W. "Effects of Physical Activity on Increased Coagulability of Blood after Ingestion of High Fat Meal." *Lancet* 2:600, 1958.

187. Mamaliga, E. *Body Development Through Weight Training.* Minneapolis: Burgess, 1976.

188. Mann, G. V. "Jogging and Coronary Heart Disease." *Circulation* 50:1283, December, 1974.

189. Matthews, D. K. *Measurement in Physical Education,* 3d ed. Philadelphia: W. B. Saunders Co., 1968.

190. Mayer, J. *A Diet for Living.* New York: David McKay Company, Inc., 1975. Consumer's Union edition, 1976.

191. ———. "Exercise and Weight Control." *Postgraduate Medicine* 25:325, 1959.

192. ——— and Bullen, B. "Nutrition and Athletic Performance." *Physiology Review* 40:369, 1960.

193. Mayhew, J. J. and Gross, P. M. "Body Composition Changes in Young Women with High Resistance Weight Training." *Research Quarterly* 45:433, 1974.

194. Martens, R. *Social Psychology and Physical Activity.* New York: Harper & Row, 1975.

195. Methany, E. *Movement and Meaning.* New York: McGraw-Hill, 1968.

196. Michele, A. A. *Orthotherapy.* New York: M. Evans & Co. Inc. 1971.

197. Miller, B. F. and Burt, J. J. *Good Health, Personal and Community.* Philadelphia: W. B. Saunders Co., 1972.

198. Miller, D. J. and Nelson, R. C. *Biomechanics of Sport.* Philadelphia: Lea & Febiger, 1973.

199. Mirken, G. "Carbohydrate Loading: A Dangerous Practice." *Journal of the American Medical Association* 233:1151, March 26, 1973.

200. Mohr, D. R. "The Contributions of Physical Activity to Skill Learning." *Research Quarterly* 31:321, 1960.

201. Morehouse, L. E. and Gross, L. *Total Fitness in 30 Minutes a Week.* New York: Simon & Schuster, 1975.

202. Morris, J. N., et al. "Vigorous Exercise in Leisure Time and Incidence of Coronary Heart Disease." *Lancet* 1:323, 1973.

203. Morrison, S. L. "Occupational Mortality in Scotland." *British Journal of Industrial Medicine* 14:130, 1957.

204. Murray, R. O. and Duncan, C. "Athletic Activity in Adolescence as an

Etiological Factor in Degenerative Hip Disease." *Journal of Bone and Joint Surgery (British)* 53:406, August, 1971.

205. Nash, J. B. *Philosophy of Recreation and Leisure.* Dubuque, Iowa: Wm. C. Brown Company Publishers, 1960.

206. Naughton, J. P., et al. *Exercise Testing and Exercise Training in Coronary Heart Disease.* New York: Academic Press, 1973.

207. Neff, W. D. *Contributions to Sensory Psychology.* New York: Academic Press, 1965.

208. Northrip, J. W., et al. *Biomechanic Analysis of Sport.* Dubuque, Iowa: Wm. C. Brown Company Publishers, 1974.

209. Ogilvie, B. and Tutko, T. "Sport: If You Want to Build Character, Try Something Else." *Psychology Today* 5:60, 1971.

210. Oscai, L. B. "The Role of Exercise in Weight Control." In *Exercise and Sports Science Reviews,* edited by J. H. Wilmore. New York: Academic Press, 1973.

211. Paffenbarger, R. S. and Hale, W. E. "Work Activity and Coronary Heart Mortality." *New England Journal of Medicine* 292:545, 1975.

212. Passwater, R. A. "Dietary Cholesterol: Is It Related to Serum Cholesterol and Heart Disease?" *American Laboratory* 44:23, September, 1972.

213. Pedley, F. G. "Coronary Disease and Occupation." *Canadian Medical Association Journal* 40:147, 1963.

214. Pipes, T. V. and Wilmore, J. H. "Isokinetic vs. Isotonic Strength Training In Adult Men." *Medicine and Science in Sports* 7:262, 1975.

215. Plagenhoef, S. *Patterns of Human Motion: A Cinematographic Analysis.* Englewood Cliffs, N. J.: Prentice-Hall, 1971.

216. Pollack, M. L., et al. "Effect of Training Two Days Per Week at Varied Intensities on Middle-Aged Men." Abstracts of Research Section of AAHPER Convention. Washington: AAHPER, 1972.

217. ———. "Effects of Walking on Body Composition and Cardiovascular Function of Middle Aged Men." *Journal of Applied Physiology* 30:126, 1971.

218. Poole, J. R. "A Cinematographic Analysis of the Upper Extremity Movements of World Class Players Executing Two Basic Badminton Strokes." *Dissertation Abstracts* 31:4531, March-April, 1971.

219. President's Council on Physical Fitness and Sports. *Adult Physical Fitness.* Washington, D. C.: U.S. Government Printing Office, publication no. 20402. Copies available from Superintendent of Documents.

220. ———. *PCPFS Newsletter.* Special Edition, May, 1973, pp. 1-27.

221. Puranen, J. "The Medial Tibial Syndrome." *Journal of Bone and Joint Surgery (British)* 56-B:712, November, 1974.

222. Raab, W. "Loafer's Heart." *Archives of Internal Medicine* 101:194, 1958.

223. Radd, A. "Statement on Physical Fitness and the Elderly." *Testimony on Physical Fitness for Older Persons.* Washington, D. C.: National Association for Human Development, 1975.

224. Ramey, M. R. "Significance of Angular Momentum in Long Jumping." *Research Quarterly* 44:488, December, 1973.

225. Rasch, P. J. "Isometric Exercise and Gains of Muscle Strength." In *Frontiers of Fitness,* edited by Roy J. Shephard. Springfield, Ill.: Charles C Thomas, Publisher, 1971, chap. 5.

226. ——— "The Present Status of Negative (Eccentric) Exercise: A Review." *American Corrective Therapy Journal* 28:77, 1974.

227. ——— and Burke, R. K. *Kinesiology and Applied Anatomy,* 4th ed. Philadelphia: Lea & Febiger, 1971.
228. Ratcliff, J. D. "Help for Your Aching Back." *Today's Health* 40:38, December, 1962.
229. Rathbone, J. and Hunt, V. *Corrective Physical Education,* 7th ed. Philadelphia: W. B. Saunders Co., 1965.
230. Riss, J. F. "Health Control Through Bio-feedback." *Modern Maturity* January, 1973, p. 67.
231. Robb, M. D. *The Dynamics of Motor Skill Acquisition.* Englewood Cliffs, N. J.: Prentice-Hall, 1972.
232. Rochmis, P. and Blackburn, H. "Exercise Tests: A Survey of Procedures, Safety and Litigation." *Journal of the American Medical Associataion* 217:1066, August 23, 1971.
233. Ryan, J. T. "A Cinematographical Analysis of the Baseball Swing." *Dissertation Abstracts* 33:4115, May, 1973.
234. Ryan, A. J. "Are You Hamstrung?" *Fitness for Living* 59, March-April, 1971.
235. ———. "Backache and What to Do About It." *Fitness for Living,* p. 78, May-June, 1970.
236. Ryan, A. J., et al. "Exercise and the Heart." *The Physician and Sports Medicine* 2:36, 1974.
237. Ryan, A. J. "Hazardous Exercises." *Fitness for Living,* p. 4, September-October, 1970.
238. ———. "What Causes Low Back Pain?" *The Physician and Sports Medicine* 2:36, 1974.
239. Sargent, J. D.; Green, E. D.; and Walters, E. D. "The Use of Autogenic Feedback Training in a Pilot Study of Migraine and Tension Headaches." A speech delivered to American Association for the Study of Headaches, July 17, 1972, San Francisco, Cal.
240. Schlesinger, Z. "Life Threatening Vagal Reaction to Physical Fitness Test." *Journal of the American Medical Association* 226:1119, November 26, 1973.
241. Schmidt, J. E. "Jogging Can Kill You." *Playboy* 23:151, March, 1976.
242. Schmidt, R. A. *Motor Skills.* New York: Harper & Row, 1975.
243. Schontz, F. C. *The Psychological Aspects of Physical Illness and Disability.* New York: Macmillan Publishing Co., Inc., 1975.
244. Schultz, J. H. and Luthe, W. *Autogenic Therapy,* vol. I. New York: Grune & Stratton, 1969.
245. Scott, M. G. and French, E. *Measurement and Evaluation in Physical Education.* Dubuque, Iowa: Wm. C. Brown Company Publishers, 1959.
246. Seltzer, C. C. and Mayer, J. "A Simple Criterion of Obesity." *Postgraduate Medicine* 38:101, 1965.
247. Selye, H. *Stress Without Distress.* Philadelphia: J. B. Lippincott Co., 1974.
248. Shaver, L. G. "Maximum Isometric Strength and Relative Muscular Endurance Gains and Their Relationships." *Research Quarterly* 42:194, 1971.
249. Sheehan, G. "Case Against Loading." *Runner's World* 11:46, August, 1976.
250. Shepard, R. J. and Kavanagh, T. "What Exercise to Prescribe for the Post-MI Patient." *The Physician and Sports Medicine* 3:57, 1975.

251. Sherrill, R. "Before You Believe Those Exercise and Diet Ads." *Today's Health* 49:34, August, 1971.

252. Sinacore, J. S. *Health: A Quality of Life*. New York: The Macmillan Co., 1968, p. 39.

253. Sloan, N. "Backaches, You Too!" *Home and Highway*, Autumn, 1964.

254. Smith, R. L. "The Bunk about Health Foods." *Today's Health* 43:24, October, 1965.

255. Soderberg, G. L. "Exercises for the Abdominal Muscles." JOHPER 37:67, September, 1966.

256. Sorenson, J. *Have Fun! Keep Fit!* Deal, N. J.: KBH Productions, 1973.

257. Stanton, G. A. "Diet and Exercise in Coronary Heart Disease." *Lancet* 2:351, August 10, 1974.

258. Stare, F. J. "Nutritional Quackery." An address presented at the Fourth National Congress on Health Quackery, October 2-3, 1968, Chicago, Illinois.

259. Steinhaus, A. *Toward an Understanding of Health and Physical Education*. Dubuque, Iowa: Wm. C. Brown Company Publishers, 1963.

260. Stevenson, J. A., et al. "Effects of Exercise on Coronary Tree Size in the Rat." *Circulation Research* 15:265, 1964.

261. Stull, G. A. and Clarke, D. H. "High-Resistance, Low-Repetition Training as a Determiner of Strength and Fatigability." *Research Quarterly* 41:189, 1970.

262. ———. "Patterns of Recovery Following Isometric and Isotonic Strength Determinant." *Medicine and Science in Sports* 3:135, 1971.

263. Stull, G. A. and Sysler, B. L. "Muscular Endurance Retention as a Function of Length of Detraining." *Research Quarterly* 41:105, 1970.

264. Swartz, F. C. "Statement on Physical Fitness and the Elderly." *Testimony on Physical Fitness for Older Persons*. Washington, D. C.: National Association for Human Development, 1975.

265. Terauds, J. "Optimal Angle of Release for the Competition Javelin as Determined By Its Aerodynamic and Ballistic Characteristics." In *Biomechanics IV*, edited by R. C. Nelson and C. A. Morehouse. Baltimore: University Park Press, 1974.

266. Thompson, H. J. *Overcoming Back Trouble*. New York: Funk and Wagnalls, 1968.

267. Thompson, H. L. "Relationship of Dynamic Balance to Speed and to Ability in Swimming." *Research Quarterly* 28:342, 1957.

268. Turner, C. E. *Personal and Community Health*. St. Louis: The C. V. Mosby Co., 1963.

269. Updyke, W. F. and Johnson, P. B. *Principles of Modern Physical Education, Health and Recreation*. New York: Holt, Rinehart and Winston, Inc., 1970.

270. Vanek, M. and Cratty, B. J. *Psychology and the Superior Athlete*. Toronto: Macmillan, 1970.

271. Van Oteghen, S. L. "Isokinetic Conditioning for Women." *Scholastic Coach* 44:87, 1974.

272. ———. "Two Speeds of Isokinetic Exercise as Related to the Vertical Jump Performance of Women." *Research Quarterly* 46:78, March, 1975.

273. Warnock, N. H.; Clarkson, T. B.; and Stevenson, R. "Effects of Exercise on Blood Coagulation Time and Atherosclerosis of Cholesterol Fed Cockerels." *Circulation Research* 5:478, 1957.

274. Wells, F. and Lutgens, K. *Kinesiology,* 6th ed. Philadelphia: W. B. Saunders Co., 1976.

275. Wheeler, R. H. and Hooley, A. M. *Physical Education for the Handicapped.* Philadelphia: Lea and Febiger, 1969.

276. Whiting, H.T.A. *Aquiring Ball Skills.* Philadelphia: Lea and Febiger, 1971.

277. Winter, A. and Winter, R., "A Pain in the Neck." *Today's Health* 46:17, June, 1968.

278. Winters, M. C. *Protective Body Mechanics: A Manual for Nurses.* Revised and edited by A. J. Bilger and E. H. Greene. New York: Springer Publishing Co., 1973.

279. Wolff, H. G., *Stress and Disease,* 2d ed. Revised and edited by S. Wolf and H. Goodell. Springfield, Ill.: Charles C Thomas, Publisher, 1968.

280. Woodworth, R. S. and Schlosberg, H. *Experimental Psychology,* 3rd ed. London: Methuen, 1972.

281. Wyrick, W. "Strength and Balance Training in Performance." *Perceptual and Motor Skills* 30:951, 1970.

282. Zuti, W. B. and Golding, L. A. "Comparing Diet and Exercise as Weight Reduction Tools." *The Physician and Sports Medicine* 4:49, 1976.

Index

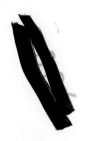